Medical Data Interpretation
for MRCP

Medical Data Interpretation for MRCP

Roger Gabriel
BA, MB, MSc, MRCP
Renal Physician
St Mary's Hospital, London

and

Cynthia M. Gabriel
MB, MRCP, DCH
Consultant Paediatrician
St. Albans City Hospital and
Queen Elizabeth II Hospital,
Welwyn Garden City, Hertfordshire

BUTTERWORTHS
London Boston
Sydney Wellington Durban Toronto

THE BUTTERWORTH GROUP

United Kingdom	**Butterworth & Co (Publishers) Ltd** **London:** 88 Kingsway, WC2B 6AB
Australia	**Butterworths Pty Ltd** **Sydney:** 586 Pacific Highway, Chatswood, NSW 2067 Also at Melbourne, Brisbane, Adelaide and Perth
Canada	**Butterworth & Co (Canada) Ltd** **Toronto:** 2265 Midland Avenue, Scarborough, Ontario, M1P 4S1
New Zealand	**Butterworths of New Zealand Ltd** **Wellington:** T & W Young Building, 77–85 Customhouse Quay, 1, CPO Box 472
South Africa	**Butterworth & Co (South Africa) (Pty) Ltd** **Durban:** 152–154 Gale Street
USA	**Butterworth (Publishers) Inc** **Boston:** 10 Tower Office Park, Woburn, Massachusetts 01801

First published 1978
Reprinted 1979

ISBN 0 407 00134 4

© Butterworth & Co (Publishers) Ltd 1978

British Library Cataloguing in Publication Data

Gabriel, Roger
  Medical data interpretation for MRCP.
  1. Diagnosis – Problems, exercises, etc
  I. Title II. Gabriel, Cynthia M
  616.07′5′076   RC71.3   78-40088

  ISBN 0-407-00134-4

Typeset by Butterworths Litho Preparation Department
Printed in England by Billings & Sons Ltd,
Guildford, London and Worcester

Contents

Preface

Passing the MRCP diploma is the entrance to serious postgraduate training. The sooner this examination has been passed the sooner the doctor can proceed with his career.

Success in examinations is in part familiarity with the kinds of questions set. We have written this book so that the MRCP candidate may practise his approach to the data section of the diploma.

We would like to thank the staff of Butterworths for their patience and assistance in producing this work.

R.G.
C.M.G.

Normal Ranges of Concentrations of Biological Substances

The normal range for biochemical and haematological concentrations varies to some extent from laboratory to laboratory. The figures quoted below are those used as normals for the purpose of this book.

BIOCHEMICAL

Plasma or serum	SI units	Conventional units
Acid phosphatase (total)	0.9–5.4 iu/l	0.5–3.0 King–Armstrong units/100 ml
Alanine transaminase (SGPT)	5–30 iu/l	
Albumin	39–45 g/l	3.9–4.5 g/100 ml
Aldosterone	100–330 pmol/l	3.5–12 ng/100 ml
Alkaline phosphatase (adults)	21–92 iu/l	3–13 King–Armstrong units/100 ml
Amylase	150–340 iu/l	80–180 Somogyi units/ 100 ml
Aspartate transaminase (SGOT)	5–30 iu/l	
Bicarbonate	22–28 mmol/l	22–28 mEq/l
Bilirubin	3–20 μmol/l	0.1–1.1 mg/100 ml
Calcium	2.25–2.6 mmol/l	9–10.5 mg/100 ml
Chloride	98–108 mmol/l	98–108 mEq/l
Cholesterol		
young adults	4.1–7.3 mmol/l	160–280 mg/100 ml
elderly	5.2–9.0 mmol/l	200–350 mg/100 ml
C3 (third component of the complement cascade)	0.1–0.18 g/l	100–180 mg/100 ml
Copper	14–22 μmol/l	17–160 μg/100 ml
Cortisol		
09.00 hours	140–700 nmol/l	5.0–25.5 μg/100 ml
24.00 hours	less than 140 nmol/l	less than 5.0 μg/100 ml

Plasma or serum	SI units	Conventional units
Creatine kinase (CPK)		
males	less than 100 iu/l	
females	less than 65 iu/l	
Creatinine		
young adults	53–133 μmol/l	0.6–1.5 mg/100 ml
elderly	70–168 μmol/l	0.8–1.9 mg/100 ml
DNA binding		less than 30%
Fibrinogen	0.2–0.4 g/l	200–400 mg/100 ml
Globulin	21–36 g/l	2.1–3.6 g/100 ml
Glucose (venous, fasting)	3.6–6.1 mmol/l	65–110 mg/100 ml
Glucose (CSF)	3.3–4.4 mmol/l	60–80 mg/100 ml
γ-Glutamyl transpeptidase		
(γ-GT)	5–30 iu/l	
Immunoglobulin G (IgG)	5–14 g/l	500–1400 mg/100 ml
Immunoglobulin A (IgA)	0.5–3.0 g/l	50–300 mg/100 ml
Immunoglobulin M (IgM)		
(adults)	0.5–2.0 g/l	50–200 mg/100 ml
Iron		
males	8–30 μmol/l	45–168 μg/100 ml
females	4–30 μmol/l	22.5–168 μg/100 ml
Iron binding capacity	45–72 μmol/l	250–400 μg/100 ml
Magnesium	0.7–0.95 mmol/l	1.4–1.9 mEq/l
Noradrenaline		
(normotensive, lying,		
Caucasian)		200–600 pg/ml plasma
5-Nucleotidase (5-NT)	4–15 iu/l	
Osmolarity	285–295 mmol/l	285–295 mmol/l
$P{CO_2}$	4.7–6.0 kPa	35–45 mmHg
$P{O_2}$	11.3–14.0 kPa	85–105 mmHg
pH	36–43 nmol/l	7.45–7.36
Phosphate (fasting)	0.7–1.4 mmol/l	2.2–4.3 mg/100 ml
Potassium	3.0–5.5 mmol/l	3.0–5.5 mEq/l
Protein (total)	62–82 g/l	6.2–8.2 g/100 ml
Protein (CSF)	0.15–0.4 g/l	15–40 mg/100 ml
Protein bound iodine	280–630 nmol/l	3.5–8.0 μg/100 ml
Renin (basal, normal sodium		
diet, normotensive)	200–2000 pg ml^{-1} h^{-1} *	
Sodium	135–146 mmol/l	135–146 mEq/l
Thyroxine (T4)	60–140 nmol/l	4.7–10.9 μg/100 ml
Triiodothyronine (T3)		
uptake**		90–117%
Triglycerides (fasting)	0.8–1.7 nmol/l	70–150 mg/100 ml
Urate† (uric acid)		
males	0.20–0.39 mmol/l	3.5–6.5 mg/100 ml
females	0.19–0.36 mmol/l	3.0–6.0 mg/100 ml
Urea†	3.3–6.6 mmol/l	20–40 mg/100 ml

* in SI units pg ml^{-1} h^{-1} is equivalent to pg/ml/h
** reduced values indicate hyperthyroidism or hypoproteinaemia
† increase in concentration with increasing age

Urine	*SI units*	*Conventional units*
Aldosterone	14–40 nmol/24 h	2–10 μg/24 h
Amylase		up to 3000 Somogyi units/24 hours
Calcium*		
males	2.5–7.5 mmol/24 h	100–300 mg/24 h
females	2.5–6.25 mmol/24 h	100–250 mg/24 h
Copper	15–78 μmol/24 h	5–25 μg/24 h
Creatinine†	9–11 mmol/24 h	1015–1245 mg/24 h
HMMA (VMA) 4-hydroxy-3-methoxy-mandelic acid	10–35 μmol/24 h	2–7 mg/24 h
Metanephrines	0.5–7.0 μmol/24 h	0.09–1.3 mg/24 h
Phosphate*	32–64 mmol/24 h	1000–2000 mg/24 h
Potassium*	30–150 mmol/24 h	30–150 mEq/24 h
Protein	less than 0.2 g/24 h	less than 200 mg/24 h
Sodium*	80–200 mmol/24 h	80–200 mEq/24 h
Urea*	250–600 mmol/24 h	15–36 g/24 h

Faeces		
Fat	11–20 mmol/24 h	3–6 g/24 h

*considerable variation with diet
† varies with muscle mass

HAEMATOLOGICAL

Plasma		
Haemoglobin		
males	13–18 g/dl	13–18 g/100 ml
females	11.5–15 g/dl	11.5–15 g/100 ml
Red blood cell count		
males	$4.5–6.5 \times 10^{12}$/l	$4.5–6.5 \times 10^{6}$/mm³
females	$3.9–5.6 \times 10^{12}$/l	$3.9–5.6 \times 10^{6}$/mm³
Packed-cell volume (PCV)		
males	0.40–0.54	40–54%
females	0.35–0.47	35–47%
Mean corpuscular haemo-globin (MCH)	27–32 pg	27–32 μμg
Mean corpuscular haemo-globin concentration (MCHC)	32–36 g/dl	32–36 g/100 ml
Mean corpuscular volume (MCV)	76–100 fl	76–100 μm³
Platelet count	$150–400 \times 10^{9}$/l	150 000–400 000/mm³
Reticulocyte count		0.2–2%
White blood cell count (WBC) (total)	$4.0–11.0 \times 10^{9}$/l	4000–11 000/mm³

Plasma	SI units	Conventional units
Differential WBC		
Neutrophils	$2.5-7.5 \times 10^9$/l	2500-7500/mm^3
Lymphocytes	$1.5-3.5 \times 10^9$/l	1500-3500/mm^3
Eosinophils	$0.04-0.44 \times 10^9$/l	40-440/mm^3
Basophils	$0.0-0.1 \times 10^9$/l	0-100/mm^3
Monocytes	$0.2-0.8 \times 10^9$/l	200-800/mm^3
Vitamin B$_{12}$	120-600 ng/l	120-600 $\mu\mu$g/ml
Folate (serum)	2.1-21 μg/l	2.1-21 ng/ml

Chapter 1

Cardiology

Question 1.1

The following figures were obtained at cardiac catheterization from an asymptomatic child aged 10 years:

Chamber	Pressure (mmHg)	Oxygen saturation (%)
Superior vena cava	–	69
Inferior vena cava	–	65
Right atrium	10	81
Right ventricle	35/0	80
Pulmonary artery	35/12	80
Left atrium	12	96
Left ventricle	105/0	95
Femoral artery	105/55	95

What was the diagnosis? ASD.

Question 1.2

The following data were obtained at cardiac catheterization from a patient aged 22 years known to have had a heart murmer from the age of 3 months:

Chamber	Pressure (mmHg)	Oxygen saturation (%)
Superior vena cava	–	69
Inferior vena cava	–	66
Right atrium	6	67
Right ventricle	120/0	66
Pulmonary artery	150/50	67
Pulmonary artery wedge	8 (mean)	–
Left ventricle	120/0	85
Aorta	120/60	85

What was the diagnosis?

Question 1.3

The following figures were obtained at cardiac catheterization from a child aged 7 years who was asymptomatic:

Chamber	Pressure (mmHg)	Oxygen saturation (%)
Superior vena cava	–	67
Inferior vena cava	–	69
Right atrium	3.5	68
Right ventricle	35/0	79
Pulmonary artery	35/10	80
Left ventricle	100/0	96

VSD   L-R

(a) What was the diagnosis?
(b) Describe the physical sign expected.

Question 1.4

A child aged 10 years was investigated by cardiac catheterization because of a heart murmur. The following data were obtained:

Chamber	Pressure (mmHg)	Oxygen saturation (%)
Superior vena cava	–	63
Inferior vena cava	–	64
Right atrium	2	86
Right ventricle	58/0	90
Pulmonary artery	17/7	89
Femoral artery	101/64	94

What was the diagnosis?   ASD ÉPS

Question 1.5

From a man aged 50 years with increasing fatigue and dyspnoea the following data were obtained at cardiac catheterization:

Chamber	Pressure (mmHg)
Right atrium	5
Right ventricle	35/9
Pulmonary artery	35/20
Pulmonary artery wedge	18
Left ventricle	210/9
Left ventricular end diastolic	22
Ascending aorta	142/70

(a) What was the diagnosis?
(b) What is the treatment?

Question 1.6

The following intra-arterial pressures were recorded from a child aged 2 years, with abnormal facies and a serum calcium of 3.27 mmol/1 (13.1 mg/100 ml):

Chamber	Pressure (mmHg)
Left ventricle	140/0
Ascending aorta	140/70
Descending aorta	85/70

What is the differential diagnosis?

Question 1.7

The following measurements were made at cardiac catheterization of a child aged 7 years who had no symptoms:

Chamber	Pressure (mmHg)	Oxygen saturation (%)
Superior vena cava	–	67
Inferior vena cava	–	69 ↓
Right atrium	3.5	68 •
Right ventricle	35/0 ↑	79 ↑
Pulmonary artery	↑35/10	80
Left ventricle	100/0	96

What was the diagnosis?   L–R at ventricular level

Question 1.8

The following data were obtained from a child aged 4 years with a 47XY karyotype:

Chamber	Pressure (mmHg)	Oxygen saturation (%)
Superior vena cava	–	66
Inferior vena cava	–	70
Right atrium	↑0	82 ↑
Right ventricle	↑50/0	83 ↑
Pulmonary artery	50/25	81 –
Left atrium	10	• 95
Left ventricle	95/0	96

What are the diagnoses?

Question 1.9

The following data were obtained during cardiac catheterization of a child aged 18 months with a history of cyanotic attacks:

Chamber	Pressure (mmHg)	Oxygen saturation (%)
Superior vena cava	–	67
Inferior vena cava	–	71
Right atrium	4	69
Right ventricle	105/6	70
Pulmonary artery	15/7	69
Left atrium	10	95
Left ventricle	105/0	84
Aorta	105/60	80

(a) What was the diagnosis?
(b) What would a postero-anterior (PA) chest X-ray show?

Question 1.10

The following pressures were obtained at cardiac catheterization from a woman aged 35 years who had a heart murmer:

Chamber	Pressure (mmHg)
Right atrium	6
Right ventricle	65/0
Pulmonary artery	65/30
Pulmonary artery wedge	18 (mean)
Left ventricle	120/0 to 120/7

(a) What was the diagnosis?
(b) What may a PA chest X-ray show?

5

Question 1.11

The following data were obtained at cardiac catheterization of a child aged 3 years:

Chamber	Pressure (mmHg)	Oxygen saturation (%)
Superior vena cava	10	45
Right atrium	10	44
Right ventricle	95/15	45
Pulmonary artery	20/10	43
Pulmonary artery wedge	15 (mean)	–
Left atrium	–	95

(a) What was the diagnosis?
(b) What feature would one expect to see on a standard chest X-ray?

Question 1.12

Seven years after a heart operation a man developed increasing fatigue, dyspnoea of exertion and paroxysmal nocturnal dyspnoea. Cardiac catheterization data:

Chamber	Pressure (mmHg)
Right atrium	13
Right ventricle	70/8
Pulmonary artery	72/38
Pulmonary artery wedge	25 (mean)
Left ventricle	155/12
Left ventricular end diastolic	9 ;
Aorta	154/80

What was the diagnosis?

Question 1.13

A man aged 45 years was admitted to hospital with a blood pressure of 230/140 mmHg and a retinopathy. Despite good control of his blood pressure fresh haemorrhages occurred in the fundi.

(*a*) Suggest three additional diagnoses.
(*b*) Suggest investigations to aid your diagnosis.

Question 1.14

A man aged 40 years developed persistent heart failure following his first myocardial infarction. There was a long systolic murmer heard over the praecordium. Investigations: Hb 11.0 g/dl (g/100 ml); MCHC 30 g/dl (g/100 ml); white blood cell count 13 × 10^9/l (13 000/mm^3); aspartate transaminase (SGOT) 25 iu/l; ECG — sinus rhythm; urine microscopy — excess of red blood cells.

(*a*) What are the differential diagnoses?
(*b*) Outline management.

Question 1.15

Following a myocardial infarction a man aged 50 years developed severe angina. Blood pressure 140/90 mmHg. Electrocardiograms showed persistent ST segment elevation in leads V3–V5. The heart was enlarged radiologically with a bulge on the left lateral border.

(*a*) What was the diagnosis?
(*b*) Outline management.

Question 1.16

A man aged 45 years was admitted to hospital after a period of crushing central chest pain. Six hours after admission the following results were available: cardiac index 1.7 litres min^{-1} m^{-2} (normal more than 3 litres min^{-1} m^{-2}); right atrial pressure 17 mmHg, total peripheral resistance 1900 dyn s/cm^5 (normal 1000–1100 dyn s/cm^5); and a blood lactate was twice normal resting concentrations.

(*a*) What was the diagnosis?
(*b*) List six likely physical signs.
(*c*) List six therapeutic measures.

7

Question 1.17

With what conditions are the following data compatible: pulse 110 beats/min; PR interval 0.22 seconds; erythrocyte sedimentation rate (ESR) 30 mm in the first hour (Westergren); ASOT 750 Todd units?

Question 1.18

Twenty-two days after an uncomplicated myocardial infarction a patient developed fever and a pericardial friction rub. Investigations: ESR 43 mm in first hour (Westergren); white blood cell count 8.1×10^9/l (8100/mm^3); neutrophils 7.3×10^9/l (7300/mm^3); lymphocytes 0.8×10^9/l (800/mm^3).

(a) What was the differential diagnosis?
(b) What additional information was necessary?

Question 1.19

A woman aged 51 years with a heart murmer had the following data: γ-globulin 50 g/l (5.0 g/100 ml); MSU — frequent red blood cells; Hb 10.8 g/dl (g/100 ml); ESR 69 mm in first hour (Westergren).

(a) What was the differential diagnosis?
(b) How may the diagnosis be established?

Question 1.20

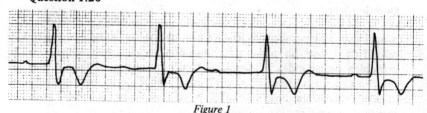

Figure 1

The above ECG trace (*Figure 1*) was taken from a left chest lead.

(a) What was the rhythm?
(b) What is the treatment?

8

Question 1.21

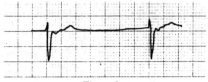

Figure 2

This trace (*Figure 2*) was taken from lead AVF recorded from a man aged 69 years taking digoxin 0.25 mg daily.

(*a*) What abnormalities were present?
(*b*) What was a probable cause?

Question 1.22

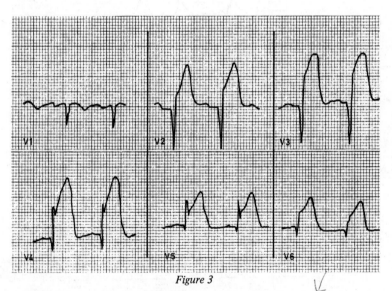

Figure 3

This ECG (*Figure 3*) was recorded from a woman aged 36 years.

(*a*) What abnormal features are present?
(*b*) What was the diagnosis?
(*c*) Suggest four predisposing factors.

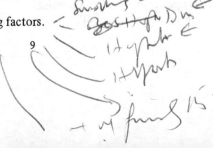

9

Question 1.23

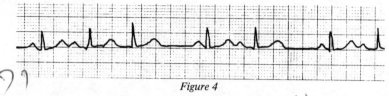

Figure 4

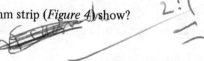

What does this rhythm strip (*Figure 4*) show?

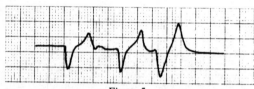

Question 1.24

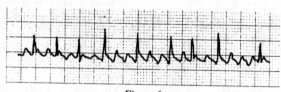

Figure 5

This rhythm strip (*Figure 5*) was taken from an ill man aged 19 years.

What does it show?

Question 1.25

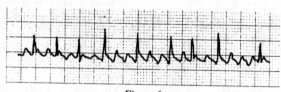

Figure 6

(a) What is this rhythm (*Figure 6*)?
(b) Suggest three underlying causes.
(c) What is the treatment?

Question 1.26

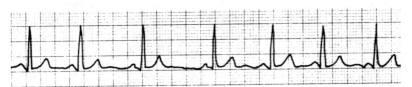

Figure 7

(a) What is this rhythm (*Figure 7*)?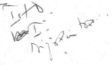
(b) State four possible causes.

Question 1.27

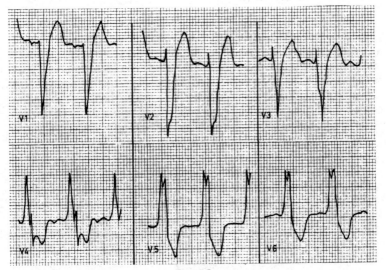

Figure 8

(a) What abnormalities do these praecordial leads show?
(b) Suggest three possible causes.

11

Question 1.28

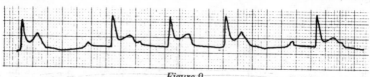

Figure 9

(*a*) What arrhythmia is this (*Figure 9*)?
(*b*) What other condition is present?

Question 1.29

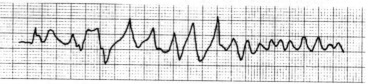

Figure 10

(*a*) What arrythmias are present (*Figure 10*)?
(*b*) What is the treatment?

Question 1.30

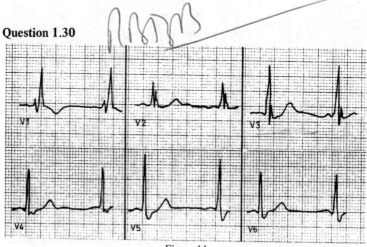

Figure 11

(*a*) What diagnoses are likely from the above chest leads (*Figure 11*)?
(*b*) Describe the abnormalities present.
(*c*) Name five possible causes.

12

Question 1.31

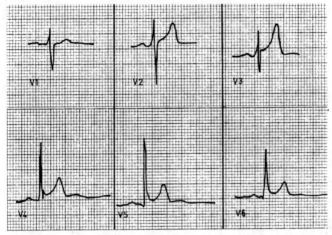

Figure 12

(*a*) What abnormalities are present in these chest leads (*Figure 12*)?
(*b*) What is the diagnosis?
(*c*) Would symptoms be present?

Question 1.32

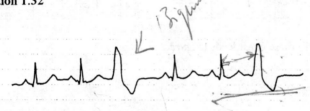

Figure 13

(*a*) What does this rhythm strip (*Figure 13*) show?
(*b*) State two possible underlying causes.

Question 1.33

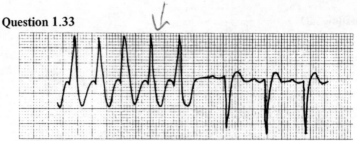

Figure 14

(*a*) What does the above trace (*Figure 14*) show?
(*b*) What simple manoeuvre changed the trace?
(*c*) What other measures are available?

Question 1.34

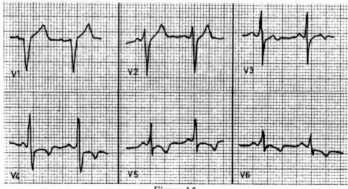

Figure 15

What do these chest leads (*Figure 15*) show?

Question 1.35

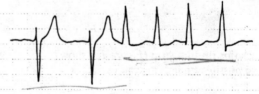

Figure 16

What does this rhythm strip (*Figure 16*) show?

14

Question 1.36

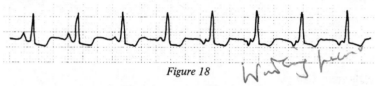

Figure 17

(*a*) What is this rhythm (*Figure 17*)?
(*b*) List six possible causes.

Question 1.37

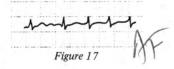

Figure 18

(*a*) What does this rhythm strip (*Figure 18*) show?
(*b*) What treatment is required?

Question 1.38

A man aged 72 years was admitted to hospital because of increasing dyspnoea. The arm to tongue time (saccharine) was 27 seconds.

What was the diagnosis?

Question 1.39

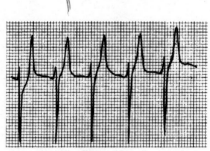

Figure 19

Is this the strip of lead V4 pathological (*Figure 19*)?

Question 1.40

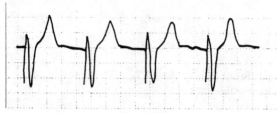

Figure 20

What does this ECG strip (*Figure 20*) show?

Question 1.41

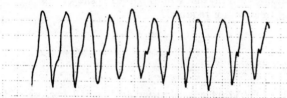

Figure 21

(*a*) What is the probable diagnosis (*Figure 21*)?
(*b*) What feature would be diagnostic?

Chapter 2
Pulmonary Disease

Question 2.1

A man aged 29 years developed an acute respiratory illness with fever and cough. Investigations: chest X-rays — right mid-zone consolidation; white blood cell count $4.0 \times 10^9/l$ ($4000/mm^3$) with a normal differential; attempts to make a blood film failed as erythrocytes agglutinated on the slide; sputum — blood stained, no bacterial pathogens cultured.

(a) What was the probable diagnosis?
(b) Suggest two tests to substantiate the diagnosis.
(c) What is the treatment?

Question 2.2

(a) What is the most common cause of the following blood-gas analysis: Po_2 55 mmHg (7.3 kPa); Pco_2 67 mmHg (9.8 kPa); pH 7.27?
(b) What figures will be found in the steady state of the same condition?

Question 2.3

A child aged 15 months presented with a history of recurrent respiratory infections. Investigations: Hb 11.0 g/dl (g/100 ml); white blood cell count 17.0 × $10^9/l$ (17 000/mm³); neutrophils 70%; lymphocytes 27%; monocytes 2%; eosinophils 1%; sweat sodium 15 mmol/l (mEq/l); serum IgA 0.30 g/l (30 mg/100 ml); IgG 9.0 g/l (900 mg/100 ml); IgM 1.5 g/l (150 mg/100 ml).

(a) What abnormalities were present?
(b) What further investigations would be appropriate?

17

Question 2.4

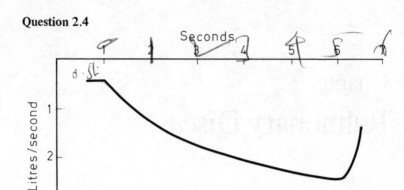

Figure 22

The above trace (*Figure 22*) was obtained from a man aged 54 years.

(*a*) With which group of diseases is the spirogram compatible?
(*b*) Explain the abnormalities.
(*c*) Is the trace compatible with normal arterial pH and blood gases?

Question 2.5

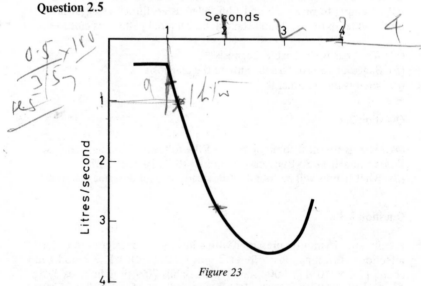

Figure 23

The above trace (*Figure 23*) was obtained from a man 183 cm tall aged 39 years.

(*a*) With what group of diseases is this spirogram compatible?
(*b*) Will the FEV_1/FVC ratio be abnormal?
(*c*) Explain the ratio.

18

Question 2.6

A man aged 42 years had the following results from lung function tests: FEV_1 2.8 litres; FVC 3.1 litres.

(a) What type of lung disease is this?
(b) Suggest a probable HLA antigen that this man might have.

Question 2.7

A baby of 35 weeks gestation, birth weight 1.9 kg had a cyanotic attack when 6 hours old. Respiratory rate was 70/min; pulse 140/min; Po_2 75 mmHg (10.0 kPa); Pco_2 50 mmHg (6.6 kPa); pH 7.15; bicarbonate 15 mmol/l (mEq/l).

(a) What was the biochemical disturbance?
(b) What was the differential diagnosis?
(c) What other investigations are essential?

Question 2.8

The following figures were obtained from an arterial blood sample taken from a patient with an acute lung complaint: Po_2 80 mmHg (10.6 kPa); Pco_2 37 mmHg (4.9 kPa); pH 7.4. After 40% inspired oxygen for 2 hours the Po_2 was 84 mmHg (11.2 kPa).

(a) What was the differential diagnosis?
(b) What is the explanation?

Question 2.9

A man of 61 years who had been previously fit developed wheezing and a productive cough. Chest X-ray — normal; peak flow rate 220 l/min; FEV_1/FVC ratio 42%; following isoprenaline inhalation FEV_1/FVC ratio 54%; sputum contained normal commensal bacteria and eosinophils.

What was the diagnosis?

19

Question 2.10

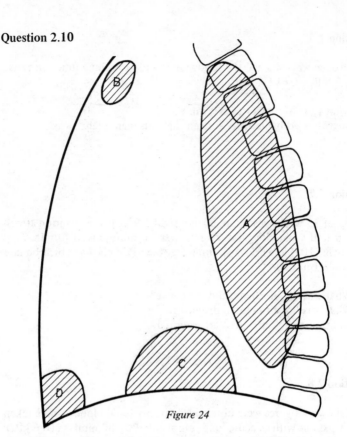

Figure 24

Figure 24 is a facsimile of a lateral view of the thorax. A, B, C and D represent areas where abnormal masses may develop.

(*a*) Name two conditions that may be found in area A.
(*b*) Name one condition that may be found in areas B, C and D.

Question 2.11

The following data were obtained by an arterial sample from a patient with a chest complaint: P_{O_2} 102 mmHg (13.6 kPa); arterial oxygen saturation 95%; P_{CO_2} 31 mmHg (4.1 kPa); pH 7.42. After exercise: P_{O_2} 77 mmHg (10.3 kPa); arterial oxygen saturation 85%; P_{CO_2} 29 mmHg (3.8 kPa); pH 7.53.

(*a*) What was the diagnosis?
(*b*) How do you explain the changes after exercise?
(*c*) What confirmatory investigations would be appropriate?

Question 2.12

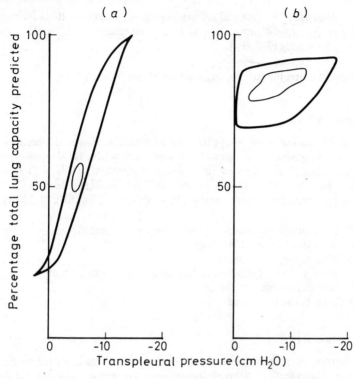

Figure 25

Figures 25(a) and (b) are pressure volume curves (lung compliance) obtained from two patients.

(a) What was the diagnosis of patient (a)?
(b) What was the diagnosis of patient (b)?

Question 2.13

A patient developed severe respiratory distress. Investigations: Po_2 53 mmHg (7.1 kPa); Pco_2 33 mmHg (4.4 kPa); pH 7.28.

With what two diagnoses are these data compatible?

Question 2.14

A woman aged 19 years had suffered recurrent chest infections for most of her life. Investigations showed: bronchiectasis; FEV_1 0.95 litres; PCO_2 58 mmHg (7.7 kPa).

Name two non-immunological tests which are indicated.

Question 2.15

A farm worker aged 34 years was admitted to hospital because of worsening episodes of cough and dyspnoea each winter for the past three years. Chest X-ray showed fine miliary infiltration; FEV_1 3.01 litres; FVC 3.5 litres; D_{CO} (T_{CO}) 10 ml min^{-1} per mmHg (predicted 25 ml min^{-1} per mmHg); PO_2 75 mmHg (10 kPa); PCO_2 25 mmHg (3.2 kPa).

(a) What additional feature in the history was essential?
(b) What was the probable diagnosis?
(c) What is the causal agent?
(d) What pattern of functional lung abnormality was present?
(e) How is this disease mediated?
(f) What is the treatment?

Question 2.16

A known chronic bronchitic of 55 years of age was admitted with an acute exacerbation. Arterial blood gases (with the patient breathing air): PO_2 50 mmHg (6.6 kPa); PCO_2 62 mmHg (8.3 kPa); bicarbonate 18 mmol/l (mEq/1); pH 7.19.

(a) Comment upon these findings.
(b) What other conditions may be present?

Question 2.17

Eight weeks after a successful renal transplant a man aged 29 years was admitted because of fever, cough and tachypnoea of 12 hours duration. Investigations: chest X-ray showed fine granular opacities throughout both lung fields; PO_2 63 mmHg (8.4 kPa); PCO_2 31 mmHg (4.2 kPa); pH 7.5.

(a) What working diagnosis should be made?
(b) What investigations are essential?
(c) What is the treatment?

Question 2.18

A coal miner aged 62 years from South Wales known to have multiple well-defined, rounded opacities in both lung fields for five years developed matudinal stiffness of the hands. Rose—Waaler test was strongly positive.

(a) What was the probable diagnosis?
(b) Is there a specific physiological defect of lung function in this condition?
(c) What is the relation of this condition to progressive massive fibrosis?

Question 2.19

At 56 hours post-hysterectomy for a cervical carcinoma an obese woman aged 59 years was noted to have a respiratory rate of 31/min. Investigations: ECG rate 120/min otherwise normal; chest X-ray showed atelectasis at the right base; Hb 9.8 g/dl (g/100 ml); Po_2 54 mmHg (7.2 kPa); Pco_2 24 mmHg (3.2 kPa); bicarbonate 30 mmol/l (mEq/l); pH 7.57.

(a) What diagnosis did the arterial sample suggest?
(b) What was the differential diagnosis?

23

Chapter 3
Gastrointestinal Disease

Question 3.1

A sample of ascitic fluid contained albumin at a concentration of 21 g/l (2.1 g/100 ml).

State three possible diagnoses.

Question 3.2

A middle-aged woman was iteric and puritic. A high titre of mitrochondrial antibodies was demonstrated in her serum.

(*a*) What was the probable diagnosis?
(*b*) What would be the histology of a biopsy of the relevant organ?

Question 3.3

A woman aged 45 years had been intermittently iteric for 9 months. Vascular spiders were present. Investigations: serum globulin 63 g/l (6.3 g/100 ml); bilirubin 49.6 μmol/l (2.9 mg/100 ml); aspartate transaminase (SGOT) 120 iu/l; alkaline phosphatase 128 iu/l (18 King–Armstrong units/100 ml); antinuclear factor (ANF) absent; DNA binding 17%; Hb$_S$Ag absent; smooth muscle antibodies present 1 in 80; mitochondrial antibodies present 1 in 10; liver biopsy showed piecemeal necrosis, prominent septa and infiltration with lymphocytes and plasma cells.

(*a*) What was the diagnosis?
(*b*) What treatment is available.

Question 3.4

After 3 months of lassitude and amenorrhoea a married woman aged 23 years was found to have the following laboratory features: Hb 13.4 g/dl (g/100 ml); white blood cell count $2.9 \times 10^9/l$ ($2900/mm^3$) with a normal differential; plasma bilirubin 100 μmol/l (5.9 mg/100 ml); alanine transaminase (SGPT) 159 iu/l; aspartate transaminase (SGOT) 390 iu/l; serum albumin 38 g/l (3.8 g/100 ml).

(*a*) What was the diagnosis from the above data?

Further investigations showed: Hb$_S$Ag absent; serum gamma globulin 60 g/l (6.0 g/100 ml); antinuclear antibody titre 1 in 1024; smooth muscle antibodies present 1 in 264; a high titre of rubella and measles antibodies.

(*b*) What was the diagnosis?
(*c*) What is the prognosis?

Question 3.5

Liver function tests showed plasma bilirubin 34 μmol/l (2.0 mg/100 ml); alkaline phosphatase 138 iu/l (19 King–Armstrong units/100 ml); aspartate transaminase (SGOT) 130 iu/l; γ-glutamyl transpeptidase 58 iu/l; serum albumin 40 g/l (4.0 g/100 ml); mitochondrial and smooth muscle antibodies positive 1 in 2.

(*a*) What do the above tests suggest?
(*b*) What would a liver biopsy be likely to show?
(*c*) Suggest causal agents.

Question 3.6

A woman aged 46 years had lost 12.3 kg in weight. Hb 10.0 g/dl (g/100 ml); ESR 17 mm in the first hour (Westergren); the ^{14}C-glycocholic acid breath test was abnormal; bilirubin 15 μmol/l (0.9 mg/100 ml); serum albumin 39 g/l (3.9 g/100 ml); Hb$_S$Ag absent; alanine transaminase (SGPT) 20 iu/l; γ-glutamyl transpeptidase 15 iu/l.

(*a*) What was the diagnosis?
(*b*) What operation had she had 5 years previously?

Question 3.7

An ill-kempt man aged 45 years of no fixed abode was brought to a casualty department by the police. He was semiconscious. Investigations: plasma sodium, potassium, chloride and bicarbonate were 130, 2.9, 71, and 40 mmol/l (mEq/l) respectively; blood urea 3.3 mmol/l (20 mg/100 ml).

(*a*) What was the diagnosis?
(*b*) Explain the biochemical findings.

Question 3.8

A life-long teetotal man aged 55 years developed discomfort over his liver two days after a myocardial infarction. Investigations: serum albumin 40 g/l (4.0 g/100 ml); alanine transaminase (SGPT) 43 iu/l, aspartate transaminase (SGOT) 51 iu/l; alkaline phosphatase 120 iu/l (17 King–Armstrong units/100 ml); serum bilirubin 34 μmol/l (2 mg/100 ml); prothrombin time 15 seconds with a control of 13 seconds.

(*a*) What was the diagnosis?
(*b*) What treatment was appropriate?

Question 3.9

A man aged 62 years had emergency abdominal surgery for colonic obstruction. Three hours postoperatively he was disproportionately ill. Investigations: Hb 15.9 g/dl (g/100 ml); white blood cell count $17 \times 10^9/l$ (17 000/mm^3); platelet count $79 \times 10^9/l$ (79 000/mm^3); plasma fibrinogen 0.05 g/l (50 mg/100 ml); fibrin degeneration products present 1 in 512; blood urea 9.7 mmol/l (64 mg/100 ml).

(*a*) What was the diagnosis?
(*b*) What are two possible complications?

Question 3.10

A man aged 58 years presented with progressive anorexia and pitting oedema. Investigations: urine normal; alkaline phosphatase 85 iu/l (12 King–Armstrong units/100 ml); alanine transaminase (SGPT) 20 iu/l; 5-nucleotidase 13 iu/l; total bilirubin 13 μmol/l (0.7 mg/100 ml); serum albumin 27 g/l (2.7 g/100 ml); BSP less than 5% retention at 45 minutes.

What is the probable explanation of these features?

Question 3.11

A man aged 40 years with coeliac disease controlled with diet developed frequent bowel actions. Faecal fat excretion was more than 20 mmol/day (more than 7 g/day).

(*a*) What were the two most likely diagnoses?
(*b*) How may these diagnoses be made?

Question 3.12

A man aged 54 years presented with dyspnoea of exertion and ascites. The blood pressure was below normal; the heart sounds were soft. Investigations: peak flow rate 480 l/min; Hb and electrolytes normal; blood urea 8 mmol/l (50 mg/100 ml); serum albumin 40 g/l (4.0 g/ 100 ml); alanine transaminase (SGPT) 45 iu/l; aspartate transaminase (SGOT) 34 iu/l; serum bilirubin 16 μmol/l (1 mg/100 ml).

What was the cause of the ascites?

Question 3.13

A woman aged 44 years was admitted to hospital with severe abdominal pain worst to the left. Paralytic ileus was present. Investigations: blood glucose 8.2 mmol/l (148 mg/100 ml); plasma bilirubin 22 μmol/l (1.3 mg/100 ml); serum calcium 1.85 mmol/l (7.4 mg/100 ml); blood urea 9.5 mmol/l (63 mg/100 ml); methaemalbuminaemia was present.

(*a*) What was the diagnosis?
(*b*) What further investigations were needed?
(*c*) What condition needed to be excluded subsequently?

Question 3.14

A man with severe dyspepsia and diarrhoea had a basal gastric acid secretion of 17 mmol of hydrogen ions in one hour. A pentagastrin test did not increase hydrogen ion secretion.

(*a*) What was the diagnosis?
(*b*) What other investigation would establish the diagnosis?
(*c*) What else should be considered in this condition?

Question 3.15

Which of the following data suggest a favourable outcome of an operation of anastomosing the portal vein to the inferior vena cava: plasma albumin 35 g/l (3.5 g/100 ml); smooth muscle antibodies 1 in 20; Alanine transaminase (SGPT) 29 iu/l; EEG normal; morphia provocation test positive; bromsulfophthalein (BSP) 9% retention at 45 minutes; $Hb_S Ag$ present?

Question 3.16

MCV (mean corpuscular volume) 110 fl(μm^3); serum calcium 2.2 mmol/l (8.8 mg/100 ml); serum albumin 38 g/l (3.8 g/100 ml).

Suggest diagnoses if these figures were obtained from:
(*a*) A Caucasian child aged 2 years.
(*b*) An Asian immigrant aged 4 years.
(*c*) A woman aged 41 years.

Question 3.17

During investigation of a gut disorder a jejunal biopsy was flat when viewed through a dissecting microscope and subtotal villous atrophy was seen histologically.

(*a*) Name two possible explanations if the patient was a Caucasian child.
(*b*) Name two explanations if the patient was an adult.

Question 3.18

A girl aged 18 months weighed 8 kg and was 75 cm high. Investigations: Hb 10.0 g/dl (g/100 ml); blood film – macrocytic; electrolytes normal; blood urea 2.9 mmol/l (17 mg/100 ml); serum calcium 2.25 mmol/l (9.0 mg/100 ml); total serum protein 50 g/l (5.0 g/100 ml); serum albumin 28 g/l (2.8 g/100 ml); xylose absorption blood taken at 30 minutes contained 15 mg/100 ml and at 60 minutes 19 mg/100 ml of D-xylose; stool tryptic activity present 1 in 50; bone age – approximately 10 months.

(*a*) What abnormalities were present?
(*b*) What further investigations were necessary?

Question 3.19

Investigation of a breast-fed baby aged 4 days showed the following: plasma bilirubin 210 μmol/l (12.3 mg/100 ml); conjugated bilirubin 20 μmol/l (1.2 mg/100 ml); blood group A Rhesus positive; Coombs' test negative; Hb 13.0 g/dl (g/100 ml); serum aspartate transaminase (SGOT) 20 iu/l; alkaline phosphatase 142 iu/l (20 King–Armstrong units/100 ml).

(*a*) What was the likely diagnosis?
(*b*) What is the differential diagnosis?
(*c*) What is the treatment?

Question 3.20

The following results were found in a jaundiced infant aged 4 weeks: total serum bilirubin 130 μmol/l (7.6 mg/100 ml); serum direct bilirubin 100 μmol/l (5.8 mg/100 ml); Hb 12 g/dl (g/100 ml); serum alkaline phosphatase 341 iu/l (48 King–Armstrong units/100 ml); serum alanine transaminase (SGPT) 40 iu/l; α-fetoprotein 56 μg/ml; prothrombin time 16 seconds, control 13 seconds.

(*a*) What were the possible diagnoses?
(*b*) How may the disease be further elucidated?

Question 3.21

A man aged 60 years underwent a technically difficult cholecystectomy. Two days postoperatively jaundice developed. On day 4 the following investigations were reported: serum bilirubin 667 μmol/l (39 mg/100 ml); serum alkaline phosphatase 19 iu/l (12.5 King–Armstrong units/100 ml); aspartate transaminase (SGOT) 75 iu/l; alanine transaminase (SGPT) 82 iu/l; $Hb_S Ag$ negative; prothrombin time 15 seconds, control 13 seconds.

Suggest two possible diagnoses.

Question 3.22

A man aged 61 years had the following blood count as an outpatient: Hb 21.5 g/dl (g/100 ml); PCV 68%; white blood cell count 12 x 10^9/l (12 000/mm^3); platelet count 570 x 10^9/l (570 000/mm^3); ESR 3 mm in the first hour. The following day he was admitted to hospital with abdominal pain and vomiting. Investigations: serum amylase 150 iu/l; alanine transaminase (SGPT) 95 iu/l; alkaline phosphatase 163 iu/l (23 King–Armstrong units/100 ml); serum albumin 36 g/l (3.6 g/100 ml); serum bilirubin 29 μmol/l (1.7 mg/100 ml); hepatic scintiscan – generally poor uptake of isotope with excess uptake in the caudate lobe.

(a) What was the primary diagnosis?
(b) What complication had occurred?
(c) What other signs would be expected to develop?
(d) What further investigation would be necessary?

Question 3.23

The following investigations were obtained from a woman aged 56 years: serum bilirubin 50 μmol/l (2.9 mg/100 ml); alanine transaminase (SGPT) 25 iu/l; serum alkaline phosphatase 772 iu/l (110 King–Armstrong units/100 ml); serum copper 161 μg/100 ml; serum ceruloplasmin 30 mg/100 ml; urine copper 85 μg/24 hours; liver copper 985 μg/g dry weight (normal 18–45 μg/g dry weight).

(a) What was the diagnosis?
(b) How might it be confirmed?

Question 3.24

An asymptomatic executive aged 40 years had a series of biochemical measurements as a routine procedure upon joining a new firm. Amongst his measurements the serum bilirubin was found to be 30 μmol/l (1.8 mg/100 ml); serum albumin 42 g/l (4.2 g/100 ml); alanine transaminase (SGPT) 15 iu/l; alkaline phosphatase 85.5 iu/l (12 King–Armstrong units/100 ml). On further investigation: the urine was seen to contain no bilirubin or urobilinogen; the reticulocyte count was 0.7%; 50% of the plasma bilirubin was unconjugated; BSP test showed less than 5% retention at 45 minutes; and a cholecystogram was normal.

(a) What was the diagnosis?
(b) Was a liver biopsy indicated?
(c) What additional test might assist in confirming the diagnosis?

Question 3.25

A woman aged 24 years with multiple ileal-ileal, ileocolic and ileo-cutaneous fistulae due to Crohn's disease was treated for 2 months with total parenteral nutrition. It was found that from time to time she developed paraesthesia, weakness and had occasional convulsions. The following investigations were reported on blood samples taken during an attack: blood urea 5.2 mmol/l (33.5 mg/100 ml); serum calcium 2.57 mmol/l (10.3 mg/100 ml); serum phosphate 0.63 mmol/l (1.9 mg/100 ml); serum albumin 34 g/l (3.4 g/100 ml); serum magnesium 0.95 mmol/l (2.28 mg/100 ml); plasma sodium 139 mmol/l; plasma potassium 2.9 mmol/l; plasma chloride 97 mmol/l; plasma bicarbonate 32 mmol/l; blood glucose 9.9 mmol/l (178 mg/100 ml); plasma choles-terol 4.1 mmol/l (158 mg/100 ml); Po_2 106 mmHg (14.1 kPa), Pco_2 37 mmHg (4.9 kPa); pH 7.45.

(a) What was the diagnosis?
(b) What was the probable cause in this woman?
(c) How may this be avoided?

Question 3.26

Explain the following figures which were obtained from a man aged 53 years: blood urea 2.2 mmol/l (13 mg/100 ml); serum calcium 1.8 mmol/l (7.2 mg/100 ml); serum albumin 27 g/l (2.7 g/100 ml); serum alkaline phosphatase 142 iu/l (20 King–Armstrong units/100 ml); Hb 9.9 g/dl (g/100 ml).

Question 3.27

A woman aged 56 years was admitted to hospital following a haema-temesis. Amongst investigations performed were the following: serum IgM 2.20 g/l (220 mg/100 ml); antimitochondrial antibodies present 1 in 60; urine pH range 6.7–7.5.

What was the diagnosis?

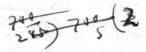

Chapter 4
Renal Disease

Question 4.1

A man aged 57 years had an emergency partial gastrectomy. The next day he was found to have a urine flow of 15 ml per hour. Investigations: electrolytes normal; blood urea 16 mmol/l (100 mg/100 ml); serum osmolarity 295 mmol/l; urine osmolarity 700 mmol/l; urine sodium 23 mmol/l (mEq/l).

Was this: dehydration; over-hydration; or acute renal failure?

Question 4.2

A man aged 21 years had a plasma creatinine of 140 μmol/l (1.6 mg/100 ml). The urine volume over a 24 hour period was 1200 ml and contained 25 mmol (2825 mg) of creatinine and 22 g of protein.

(a) What was the creatinine clearance?
(b) How do you explain this value?

Question 4.3

A patient with nephrotic syndrome has the following: daily weight gain of 0.5 kg; plasma volume reduced by 17%; selectivity of proteinuria 0.01; urine calcium excretion 0.3 mmol/day (12 mg/day); serum cholesterol 20.4 mmol/l (790 mg/100 ml); serum albumin 27 g/l (2.7 g/100 ml); serum C3 0.035 g/l (35 mg/100 ml); plasma aldosterone 990 pmol/l; urine protein excretion varying between 12 and 19 g/day; the presence of purpura; a blood pressure of 150/115 mmHg. Which of the above are prognostically significant in:

(a) A child aged 5 years?
(b) An adult?

Question 4.4

Urine obtained from bilateral ureteric catheters contained the following:

	Catheter A	Catheter B
Urine volume (ml/min)	2.9	0.6
Urine sodium (mmol (mEq)/min)	0.2	0.08
Urea (mmol/min)	0.19	0.35
(mg/min)	1.09	2.1
Para-aminohippurate (mg/ml)	0.7	2.9

What was the diagnosis? *RAS*

Question 4.5

From a man aged 59 years the following results became available: 24 hour urine 12–15 g protein; protein selectivity 0.7; 24 hour glucose excretion 9–11 g.

K.W. Syndrome

What was the probable diagnosis?

Question 4.6

A boy aged 5 years presented with anasarca of 4 days duration. The plasma albumin was 23 g/l (2.3 g/100 ml) and the urine protein selectivity was 0.01.

minimal change. Nephrotic Syndrome

(a) What was the diagnosis?
(b) What is the treatment?
(c) What was the chance of remission with or without treatment?

Question 4.7

From a patient with chronic bone disease the following data were available: serum calcium 2.0 mmol/l (8 mg/100 ml); alkaline phosphatase 270 iu/l (38 King–Armstrong units/100 ml); 25–OHD$_3$ normal, 1, 25-di-OHD$_3$ and 24, 25-di-OHD$_3$ 20–30% of standard reference sera; parathyroid hormone — more than upper limit of assay.

Renal Osteo dystrophy

(a) What was the bone disease?
(b) What is the explanation?
(c) Suggest what the serum inorganic phosphate and urate would be if measured at the same time.

Question 4.8

A Caucasian aged 13 years developed haematuria. At cystoscopy the bladder was normal. Investigations: urine microscopy — granular and red cell casts, sterile on culture; GFR 118 ml/min (corrected for surface area); protein excretion 0.2 g/day; serum IgA 158% of normal reference sera; ASOT 150 Todd units.

(*a*) Suggest two possible diagnoses.
(*b*) What additional features of history were needed?

Question 4.9

The following measurements were made in a girl aged 19 years with dependent pitting oedema: urine protein excretion 11.5 g/12 hours; urine sodium 8 mmol (mEq) per litre per 12 hours; plasma sodium 139 mmol/l (mEq/l); plasma potassium 4.2 mmol/l (mEq/l); serum albumin 23 g/l (2.3 g/100 ml); serum cholesterol 22 mmol/l (851 mg/100 ml); urine microscopy — granular casts and epithelial cells; culture of urine — sterile.

(*a*) With what condition are these findings compatible?
(*b*) What will be the urinary aldosterone excretion?

Question 4.10

With what conditions are the following electrolytes associated: plasma sodium 140 mmol/l (mEq/l); plasma chloride 109 mmol/l (mEq/l); plasma bicarbonate 15 mmol/l (mEq/l); plasma potassium 3.0 mmol/l (mEq/l)?

Question 4.11

A woman aged 23 years had unilateral renal disease and hypertension. Investigations: glomerular filtration rate (GFR) 72 ml/min; urine protein excretion 2.1 g/day; urine sterile for Gram-staining bacteria and acid-fast bacteria; peripheral venous renin 1.9; right renal venous renin 2.1; left renal venous renin 4.7 (renin expressed as ng ml^{-1} mm^{-1}).

(*a*) What renal disease was present?
(*b*) Was a nephrectomy indicated?

Question 4.12

Blood urea 14.5 mmol/l (96 mg/100 ml); serum creatinine 395 μmol/l (4.5 mg/100 ml).

(a) Comment upon the above data.
(b) Name three conditions in which they may be found.

Question 4.13

Which of the following would be of help in the differentiation of acute from chronic renal failure in a man aged 40 years: Hb 11.9 g/dl (g/100 ml); blood urea 27.5 mmol/l (182 mg/100 ml); plasma creatinine 985 μmol/l (11.1 mg/100 ml); serum urate 0.65 mmol/l (10.9 mg/ 100 ml); serum calcium 2.01 mmol/l (8.0 mg/100 ml); serum phosphate 2.95 mmol/l (9.1 mg/100 ml); serum magnesium 0.68 mmol/l (1.36 mg/ 100 ml); serum albumin 39 g/l (3.9 g/100 ml); U/P osmolarity 1.5 (urine flow 1 ml/min); plasma glucose 6.9 mmol/l (124 mg/100 ml); plasma bilirubin 16 μmol/l (0.9 mg/100 ml); fasting cholesterol 9.1 mmol/l (352 mg/100 ml); fasting triglyceride 4.9 mmol/l (434 mg/ 100 ml)?

Question 4.14

Which of the following investigations would aid in the differentiation between a patient with early (a few hours) acute renal failure and a patient with long-standing chronic renal failure receiving a 30 g protein diet: haemoglobin; blood urea; plasma sodium; plasma potassium; serum calcium; serum phosphate?

Question 4.15

A girl aged 18 years with mild oedema had the following findings: blood urea 19.5 mmol/l (128 mg/100 ml); serum albumin 29 g/l (2.9 g/100 ml); urine protein excretion 5–10 g/day. h - s

(a) What was the diagnosis?

Two weeks later her weight had increased by 15 kg. Urine – sterile; protein excretion 25–30 g/day; blood urea 42.8 mmol/l (282 mg/100 ml); serum albumin 21 g/l (2.1 g/100 ml).

(b) What was the probable diagnosis at that stage? RVT
(c) Outline management.

Question 4.16

A man aged 25 years was reported to have had glycosuria. The following glucose tolerance test (GTT) was obtained:

Time (min)	Glucose (mmol/l)	(mg/100 ml)
0	4.7	85
30	6.3	113
60	9.8	176
90	6.2	112
120	5.4	97

What may be the diagnosis?

Question 4.17

A patient's blood urea rose from 18.8 mmol/l (113 mg/100 ml) to 35.6 mmol/l (214 mg/100 ml) in 24 hours.

Suggest three causes.

Question 4.18

The following data were obtained from a woman aged 27 years with 'cystitis': PCV 49%; plasma sodium 140, plasma potassium 7.5, plasma bicarbonate 27, plasma chloride 101 mmol/l (mEq/l); serum calcium 2.55 mmol/l (10.2 mg/100 ml); serum phosphate 0.7 mmol/l (2.2 mg/100 ml).

What was abnormal and what is the probable explanation?

Question 4.19

In an adult, bilateral nephrocalcinosis was found in association with: osteoid border greater than 15 μm; urine calcium 2.1 mmol/day (84 mg/day); arterial pH 7.31; urinary pH 5.4.

What is the differential diagnosis?

36

Question 4.20

A patient who had received a transplant kidney 35 days previously developed a flu-like illness. Investigations: Hb 10.7 g/dl (g/100 ml); white blood cell count 20 × 10^9/l (20 000/mm^3), neutrophils 18 000, lymphocytes 1400, monocytes 200, eosinophils 400; platelets 100 × 10^9/l (100 000/mm^3); 24 hour urine volume 780 ml; creatinine clearance 43 ml/min; urine protein excretion 4.7 g/l.

(a) What was the likely diagnosis?
(b) Name six other features of this condition.

Question 4.21

A man aged 65 years presented with haematuria. Investigations: urine — sterile; intravenous pyelogram (IVP) — mass arising from lower pole of left kidney with calyceal distortion; alkaline phosphatase 156 iu/l (22 King–Armstrong units/100 ml); BSP retention test — 17% retained at 45 minutes; isotope scan of liver — normal.

What was the diagnosis?

Question 4.22

A schoolboy aged 16 years took a constant diet containing 120 mmol (mEq) of sodium, 100 mmol (mEq) potassium and 24.25 mmol (970 mg) of calcium daily. On the fifth day of the diet the urine volume was 950 ml and contained 8 mmol (mEq) sodium, 70 mmol (mEq) potassium and 0.25 mmol (10 mg) calcium; urinary urea was 423 mmol (25.5 g); and urinary creatinine was 14.5 mmol (1640 mg). The IVP showed enlarged symmetrical kidneys.

(a) Suggest two diagnoses.
(b) Explain the urinary electrolytes.
(c) Suggest a further important urinary measurement which is needed.

Question 4.23

The following measurements were made on a 'random' urine sample from a patient who had recently become oliguric: sodium 92 mmol/l (mEq/l); osmolarity 312 mmol/l; urea concentration 75 mmol/l (450 mg/100 ml); Blood taken at the same time showed: plasma sodium 142 mmol/l (mEq/l); plasma potassium 5.3 mmol/l (mEq/l); plasma bicarbonate 23 mmol/l (mEq/l); blood urea 10.8 mmol/l (65 mg/100 ml); osmolarity 288 mmol/l.

(a) What was the diagnosis?
(b) Would the patient respond with a diuresis to intravenous saline and a 'loop' diuretic?
(c) What would a high dose IVP probably show?

Question 4.24

A Caucasian man aged 29 years was found to have a blood pressure of 170/115 mmHg. Plasma renin was 37 pg ml^{-1} h^{-1} and plasma aldosterone 1590 pmol/l. He was given a 10 mmol (mEq) diet for 5 days. At the end of this period the plasma renin and plasma aldosterone were 42 pg ml^{-1} h^{-1} and 1630 pmol/l respectively.

(a) What was the diagnosis?
(b) Name one further essential investigation.
(c) What is the treatment?

Question 4.25

A normotensive medical student participating in a metabolic experiment took diet A for one week. His recumbent plasma renin was then 1700 pg per ml plasma per hour and the plasma aldosterone was 590 pmol/l. Diet B was then given for 7 days after which recumbent plasma renin was 670 pg ml^{-1} h^{-1} and plasma aldosterone was 195 pmol/l.

(a) What was the approximate sodium content of diets A and B?
(b) With reference to the sodium intake and assuming other constituents of the diet were kept constant what difference in urine volume and urine sodium would you expect at the end of the first and the second weeks?

Question 4.26

During the investigation of a proteinuria of 1.3 g/day in a man aged 40 years the following results were obtained: plasma pH 7.35 (45 nmol/l); persistent glycosuria; uric acid clearance 14.5 ml/min; plasma phosphate 0.5 mmol/l (1.55 mg/100 ml); maximum urine acidity after 0.1 g/kg bodyweight load of ammonium chloride 5.9; maximum urinary concentration after dehydration and pitressin 499 mmol/l; chromotography of urine – generalized amino-aciduria; electrophoresis of urine protein – little albumin and increased quantities of β-microglobulin.

(a) What was the diagnosis?
(b) What type of curve would be obtained if a GTT were performed in this man?

Question 4.27

A woman aged 21 years was admitted with an inevitable abortion and a D and C was performed for necrotic infected retained products. Postoperatively the urine was red/black in colour. Investigations: Hb 8.2 g/dl (g/100 ml); white blood cell count 25 × 10^9/l (25 000/mm^3); neutrophils 87%; lymphocytes 13%; reticulocyte count 8%; indirect plasma bilirubin 94 μmol/l (5.5 mg/100 ml); platelets 75 × 10^9/l (75 000/mm^3).

(a) What were the diagnoses?
(b) What are probable complications?

Question 4.28

A woman aged 48 years presented with polydipsia and polyuria of 3 months' duration. Investigations: urine volume 5–8.5 l/day; blood urea 5 mmol/l (30 mg/100 ml); mean of 5 measurements of plasma osmolarity 285 mmol/l; following intramuscular pitressin urine volume fell to 4.5 in 24 hours but polydipsia continued.

What was the diagnosis?

Question 4.29

A man aged 40 years had progressive back and pelvic girdle discomfort. Investigations: X-ray of spine – 'cod fish' vertebrae; X-ray of abdomen – nephrocalcinosis of medullary distribution; urine pH 7.0–6.4; 3 days' faecal fat excretion 13.5 mmol/day (3.8 g/day); D-xylose absorption 1.1 g excreted in 5 hours after 5 g orally; blood urea 5.5 mmol/l (33 mg/100 ml); serum calcium 2.0 mmol/l (8 mg/100 ml); serum phosphate 1.4 mmol/l (4.3 mg/100 ml); serum albumin 41 g/l (4.1 g/100 ml); arterial pH 7.3.

(a) What were the diagnoses?
(b) What confirmatory test was indicated?

Question 4.30

A girl aged 17 years taking her usual Western European diet had a urinary sodium of 90–110 mmol (mEq) daily. Her recumbent plasma renin activity was 87 pg per ml plasma per hour and urinary aldosterone was 22 μg/24 h. She was then given 0.2 mg of 9 α-fluorohydrocortisone twice daily for three days and did not change her diet. At the end of this period the recumbent plasma renin activity was 29 pg ml^{-1} h^{-1}; the plasma aldosterone was 90 pmol/l; and the urinary aldosterone 13 μg/24 h.

What do these findings suggest?

Question 4.31

With what conditions are the following data compatible: glycosuria; creatinine clearance 159 ml/min; urea 2.5 mmol/l (15 mg/100 ml)?

Question 4.32

A man aged 51 years took medical advice because of two episodes of haematuria. The blood pressure was 175/122 mmHg. Investigations: urea 5.9 mmol/l (35 mg/100 ml); plasma electrolytes normal; urine microscopy – epithelial cells only; urine culture – sterile. The blood pressure was successfully treated. Two months later he felt unwell and was reinvestigated: urea 32.1 mmol/l (193 mg/100 ml); plasma sodium 130, potassium 5.5, bicarbonate 16 mmol/l (mEq/l); urine microscopy – many erythrocytes and white blood cells; no casts, urine culture sterile;

IVP – poor opacification and dilatation of right renal pelvis, left kidney not demonstrated; total serum acid phosphatase 6.5 iu/l (3.6 King–Armstrong units/100 ml).

(*a*) What was the probable diagnosis?
(*b*) What urgent investigation was needed?
(*c*) Comment upon initial management.

Question 4.33

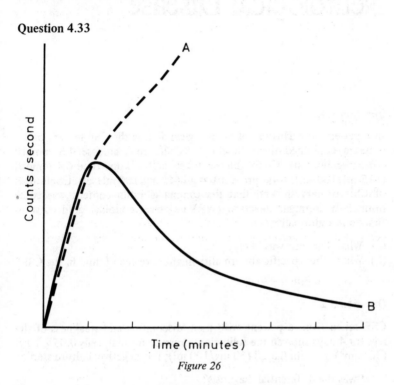

Figure 26

A patient presented with sudden severe loin pain and renogram trace A (*Figure 26*) was found. A renal operation was performed and 3 weeks later trace B was recorded. The following month a further operation remote from the kidney was performed.

(*a*) What does trace A show?
(*b*) What operation was first performed?
(*c*) What does trace B show?
(*d*) What was the second operation?
(*e*) Name three relevant investigations indicating the need for the second operation.

41

Chapter 5
Neurological Disease

Question 5.1

In a patient with a history of neurological disease the CSF under normal pressure contained the following: 1 cell/2 hpf; glucose 4.3 mmol/l (77.5 mg/100 ml), blood glucose taken at the same time 6.4 mmol/l (115 mg/100 ml); total protein 0.4 g/l (40 mg/100 ml); electrophoresis of CSF protein showed that the gamma globulin content was twice normal; Wassermann reaction (WR) negative; colloidal gold curve — first-zone abnormality.

(a) What diagnosis was likely?
(b) What other specific abnormality might have been found in the CSF?

Question 5.2

CSF taken from a patient with pain, discomfort and weakness of the legs for 4 days showed the following: pressure normal; cells $0.05 \times 10^9/l$ (50/mm³); protein 0.5 g/l (50 mg/100 ml); WR negative; culture sterile.

What was the differential diagnosis?

Question 5.3

A baby aged 4 months was found to have poor head control and generalized hypotonia. A detailed perinatal history was not available. Occipital—frontal circumference 38.5 cm; weight 6.4 kg; length 63 cm; birth weight 3.0 kg.

(a) Comment on the data.
(b) Suggest possible explanations.
(c) List investigations into the aetiology.

Question 5.4

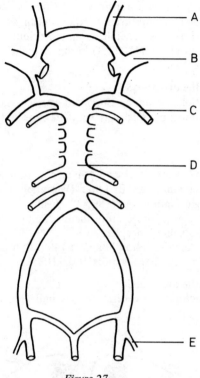

Figure 27

What are the vessels A, B, C, D and E and what lesion will result from the occlusion of each (*Figure 27*)?

Question 5.5

A Caucasian patient with Cushing's disease was treated by bilateral adrenalectomy. Three years later he returned to the clinic complaining of increasing deterioration of vision. Plasma adrenocorticotrophic hormone (ACTH) concentration was 4500 pg/ml.

(*a*) What was the diagnosis?
(*b*) What sign will probably be very obvious?
(*c*) What neurological signs could be expected to be found?
(*d*) What is the treatment?

Question 5.6

A boy aged 14 years with a history of a Coombs' negative haemolytic anaemia developed a mixture of Parkinsonism and cerebellar ataxia. Investigations showed a generalized amino aciduria; glycosuria; serum urate 100 μmol/l (1.7 mg/100 ml); serum copper 90 μg/100 ml; urine copper 2300 μg/24 h.

(*a*) What was the diagnosis?
(*b*) What additional serum measurement was necessary?
(*c*) What additional physical sign would be expected to be found?

Question 5.7

A man aged 67 years developed tender and painful muscles. Investigations: ESR 41 mm in the first hour (Westergren); ANF positive 1:10; sheep cell agglutination test (SCAT) positive 1:4; serum bilirubin 15 μmol/l (0.9 mg/100 ml); serum alanine transaminase (SGPT) 52 iu/l; LDH 420 iu/l; alkaline phosphatase 85 iu/l (12 King–Armstrong units/100 ml); serum creatine phosphokinase 149 iu/l; total acid phosphatase 9.5 iu/l (5.3 King–Armstrong units/100 ml).

(*a*) What was the diagnosis?
(*b*) What neurological investigation was indicated and what would it demonstrate?

Question 5.8

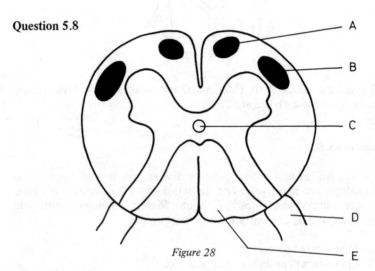

Figure 28

Figure 28 shows a cross-section of the spinal cord. What will lesions at sites A, B, C, D and E produce?

Question 5.9

A baby was noted to have a head circumference of 44 cm at 3 months of age and a weight of 6.3 kg. At birth the head circumference had been 35.5 cm and the weight 3.5 kg.

(*a*) What abnormalities were present?
(*b*) What are the possible causes?
(*c*) What clinical features might be expected?
(*d*) What investigations were required?

Question 5.10

Intracranial calcification was seen on the X-ray of a child aged 4 years. The occipital frontal circumference was 48 cm.

List possible causes.

Question 5.11

A woman aged 29 years with a 17 week singleton pregnancy had a serum α-fetoprotein 2.7 times greater than was normal for a comparable woman at that stage of pregnancy.

(*a*) What was the possible diagnosis?
(*b*) What further investigations were necessary?
(*c*) What other cause of raised α-fetoprotein is there?

Question 5.12

The CSF from a patient with a maculopapular reddish rash showed the following: pressure – moderately raised; cells $0.2 \times 10^9/l (200/mm^3)$ predominantly lymphocytes; protein 0.45 g/l (45 mg/100 ml); glucose 3.9 mmol/l (17 mg/100 ml); bacteriological culture sterile.

What is the differential diagnosis?

Question 5.13

An EEG from a child showed a 3/s generalized wave and spike activity.

(*a*) What was the diagnosis?
(*b*) What symptoms would be expected during the recording of the described EEG?

Question 5.14

A woman aged 20 years was admitted because of anxiety depression and a facial rash. There were no focal neurological signs. Investigations: Hb 13.2 g/dl (g/100 ml); white blood cell count 5.0 × 10^9/l (5000/mm^3), neutrophils 88%, eosinophils 2%, monocytes 1%, lymphocytes 9%. The EEG showed diffused non-specific findings. Serum C3 29% of normal; DNA binding 70%.

(*a*) What was the diagnosis?
(*b*) What is the treatment?

Question 5.15

From a child aged 13 months the following CSF findings were reported: white cell content 250/hpf, 90% neutrophils; protein concentration 1.0 g/l (100 mg/100 ml); glucose 2.1 mmol/l (38 mg/100 ml); the peripheral blood glucose measured from blood taken immediately after the lumbar puncture was 6.2 mmol/l (111 mg/100 ml).

(*a*) What was the diagnosis?
(*b*) What will be the major immunoglobulin constituent of the CSF protein?
(*c*) What additional urgent information may be obtained from the CSF?
(*d*) What is the treatment?

Question 5.16

A woman aged 49 years presented with earache, deafness and dribbling. A left lower motor neuron of the seventh nerve and left nerve deafness were present. There were vesicles on the ear, external auditory meatus and soft palate. Investigations: Hb 9.8 g/dl (g/100 ml); white blood cell count normal; blood film roleaux present; ESR 72 mm in the first hour (Westergren); electrolytes normal; serum albumin 40 g/l (4.0 g/100 ml); alanine transaminase (SGPT) 60 iu/l; gamma globulin 61 g/l (6.1 g/100 ml).

(*a*) What was the cause of her symptoms?
(*b*) What was the cutaneous nerve supply of the area involved?
(*c*) What further investigations were indicated?

Question 5.17

CSF taken from a child who had become progressively unwell for 10 days contained the following: 0.17 cells $\times$ $10^9/l$ (170/mm^3) which were approximately half lymphocytes and half neutrophils; protein concentration 1.55 g/l (155 mg/100 ml); glucose 1.9 mmol/l (34 mg/100 ml); Gram stain of CSF — no organisms found.

(*a*) What was the probable diagnosis?
(*b*) What other investigations were needed?

Question 5.18

A 4-day-old baby, birth weight 2.8 kg was noted to have a convulsion. Investigations: blood glucose 1.7 mmol/l (30 mg/100 ml); serum calcium 2.0 mmol/l (8.0 mg/100 ml); prothrombin time 14 seconds with a control of 13 seconds; plasma sodium 135, potassium 4.0, bicarbonate 20 mmol/l (mEq/l); urea 4.1 mmol/l (35 mg/100 ml).

(*a*) What was the probable diagnosis?
(*b*) What further investigations should have been undertaken?

Question 5.19

What is the differential diagnosis of an adult patient with a central venous pressure of +10 to 15 cmH$_2$O, a cardiac output of 1.4 l/min and a motor conduction time of 20 m/s?

Question 5.20

A patient had neurological signs in the legs. CSF showed the following: colour xanthochromic; pressure 14 cmH$_2$O; protein 4.9 g/l (490 mg/100 ml); glucose 4.05 mmol/l (7.3 mg/100 ml); cells 2 lymphocytes/mm^3; culture was reported as sterile.

(*a*) What was the diagnosis?
(*b*) What was the differential diagnosis?

Chapter 6
Metabolic Conditions

Question 6.1

A woman aged 62 years had persistent vomiting. Investigations: barium meal normal; blood urea 29 mmol/l (175 mg/100 ml); serum calcium 3.8 mmol/l (13.5 mg/100 ml); serum phosphate 1.8 mmol/l (5.5 mg/100 ml); alkaline phosphatase 71 iu/l (10 King–Armstrong units/100 ml); serum albumin 40 g/l (4.0 g/100 ml); Hb 9.7 g/dl (g/100 ml).

(*a*) What was the cause of the vomiting?
(*b*) Suggest two diagnoses.

Question 6.2

What conditions may produce the following electrolyte changes: sodium 132, chloride 88, potassium 3.1 mmol/l (mEq/l); serum calcium 3.0 mmol/l (12.1 mg/100 ml).

Question 6.3

A baby aged 9 months presented with crying and refusal of feeds for 24 hours. There was generalized swelling of the lower face. Rectal temperature 38.5°C. Investigations: Hb 9.8 g/dl (g/100 ml); blood film normocytic; white blood cell count 30 × 10^9/l (30 000/mm^3) with 80% neutrophils; ESR 40 mm in the first hour (Westergren); random urine protein excretion 0.2 g/l (200 mg/100 ml).

(*a*) What was the differential diagnosis?
(*b*) What further investigations were indicated?

Question 6.4

A man aged 75 years who lived alone in a single room complained of increasing back and pelvic discomfort for 18 months. Investigations: creatinine clearance 68 ml/min; serum calcium 2.0 mmol/l (8 mg/100 ml); serum inorganic phosphate 0.6 mmol/l (1.9 mg/100 ml); serum urate 0.4 mmol/l (6.7 mg/100 ml); alkaline phosphatase 127 iu/l (19 King–Armstrong units/100 ml); urine calcium 5.0 mmol/24 h (200 mg/24 h).

(a) What was the probable diagnosis?
(b) What additional investigations were needed?
(c) What treatment is necessary?

Question 6.5

Blood glucose 4.2 mmol/l (75 mg/100 ml); plasma sodium 131 mmol/l (mEq/l).

Name three conditions compatible with these findings.

Question 6.6

A man aged 46 years with long-standing back disease had the following investigations: serum calcium 2.6 mmol/l (10.4 mg/100 ml); serum phosphate 1.6 mmol/l (3.72 mg/100 ml); alkaline phosphatase 78 iu/l (11 King–Armstrong units/100 ml); serum urate 0.47 mmol/l (7.9 mg/100 ml); B27 HLA (human leucocyte antigen) present; blood urea 7.9 mmol/l (52 mg/100 ml).

(a) What was the diagnosis?
(b) What would X-ray of the spine show?
(c) If there were a heart murmur in this patient what would one expect the pulse pressure to be?

Question 6.7

A man was admitted at a relatively early stage of an illness before any therapy had been given. Investigations: blood volume 68 ml/kg body-weight; plasma renin 400 ng ml^{-1} h^{-1}; plasma aldosterone 457 pmol/ml.

Name three illnesses compatible with the above data.

Question 6.8

Are the following figures compatible with a plasma osmolarity of 290 mmol/l: plasma sodium 150, chloride 106 mmol/l (mEq/l); serum calcium 2.6 mmol/l (10.4 mg/100 ml); serum phosphate 1.5 mmol/l (4.6 mg/100 ml); serum albumin 44 g/l (4.4 g/100 ml); blood urea 7.2 mmol/l (47 mg/100 ml); blood glucose 5.2 mmol/l (94 mg/100 ml); plasma potassium 4.0 mmol/l (mEq/l)?

Question 6.9

Comment upon the following figures obtained from a man aged 47 years: serum creatinine 123 μmol/l (1.4 mg/100 ml); liver function – normal; total serum protein 60 g/l (6.0 g/100 ml); serum albumin 30 g/l (3.0 g/100 ml); serum urate 0.55 mmol/l (9.2 mg/100 ml); serum calcium 2.7 mmol/l (10.8 mg/100 ml); serum phosphate 1.1 mmol/l (3.4 mg/100 ml); serum cholesterol 8.4 mmol/l (325 mg/100 ml); serum triglyceride 1.95 mmol/l (173 mg/100 ml).

Question 6.10

Blood taken from a man contained urea at a concentration of 15.2 mmol/l (91 mg/100 ml) and creatinine at 133 μmol/l (1.5 mg/100 ml).

Suggest five explanations for the discrepancy.

Question 6.11

A previously healthy man aged 49 years presented with heart failure. Investigations: Hb 14.6 g/dl (g/100 ml); PCV 51%; white blood cell count 10 × 10⁹/l (10 000/mm³), 82% of which were neutrophils; fasting blood glucose 11 mmol/l (198 mg/100 ml); serum albumin 39 g/l (3.9 g/100 ml); serum alanine transaminase (SGPT) 132 iu/l; serum iron 62.5 μmol/l (350 μg/100 ml); iron binding capacity 70 μmol/l (329 μg/100 ml).

(a) What was the diagnosis?
(b) List four further clinical features of this condition.

Question 6.12

The following measurements were made in an ill patient: BP 90/50 mmHg; pulse 120 per min; arterial pH 7.22, Po_2 63 mmHg (8.4 kPa); Pco_2 34 mmHg (4.5 kPa); blood lactate 5.9 mmol/l; urine pH 5.2; urine osmolarity 320 mmol/l; blood glucose 8.4 mmol/l (152 mg/100 ml).

(a) What was the diagnosis?
(b) What underlying conditions could have been present?
(c) May drugs cause this condition?
(d) What is the treatment?

Question 6.13

Following a herniorrhaphy a man aged 68 years developed a tender swollen knee joint. Investigations: ESR 42 mm in the first hour (Westergren); white blood cell count 13.0×10^9/dl (13 000 mm^3) with 79% neutrophils; blood urea 9.9 mmol/l (59 mg/100 ml); serum urate 0.56 mmol/l (9.5 mg/100 ml). Aspiration of the joint fluid showed weak positive birefringence of crystals within a neutrophil.

What was the diagnosis?

Question 6.14

A 19-year-old Asian immigrant recently arrived in Britain had headaches for 6 weeks and was found unrousable one morning. Investigations: Hb 15.1 g/dl (g/100 ml); white blood cell count 14.9 x 10^9/l (14 900/ mm^3) with 77% neutrophils; plasma sodium 150, potassium 4.9, bicarbonate 11 mmol/l (mEq/1); blood urea 13.6 mmol/l (82 mg/100 ml); plasma osmolarity 353 mmol/l; urine osmolarity 770 mmol/l; CSF faintly opalescent and under increased pressure; protein 2.1 g/l (210 mg/100 ml); glucose concentration 17.9 mmol/l (322 mg/100 ml); cell count 0.2 × 10^9/l (200/mm^3) chiefly of neutrophils; Gram stain of CSF — no organisms seen.

(a) What was the blood glucose concentration?
(b) What was the diagnosis?
(c) Comment on the serum and urine osmolarities.

Question 6.15

A man aged 72 years attended his doctor because of a sudden pain in the right great toe joint. Investigations: Hb 13.0 g/dl (g/100 ml); ESR 17 mm in the first hour (Westergren); electrolytes normal; urea 8.2 mmol/l (49 mg/100 ml); serum urate 0.54 mmol/l (9.0 mg/100 ml); ANF positive 1 in 10.

What was the diagnosis?

Question 6.16

In a man aged 40 years fasting plasma stored for 12 hours at 4°C was turbid and had a creamy layer. Cholesterol concentration 12.5 mmol/l (485 mg/100 ml); triglyceride 8.7 mmol/l (770 mg/100 ml); electrophoresis of the lipoproteins showed an abnormal β-lipoprotein.

(*a*) What type of hyperlipidaemia was this?
(*b*) Name three associated conditions.
(*c*) What treatment is usually recommended?

Question 6.17

A full-term baby, birth weight 2.8 kg became jaundiced at 36 hours. On the eighth post-delivery day she weighed 2.45 kg and showed bruising. Investigations: mother's blood group 0 negative; infant's blood group A positive; total bilirubin 136 μmol/l (7.9 mg/100 ml); Hb 15 g/dl (g/100 ml); prothrombin time 16 seconds with a control of 13 seconds; platelet count 180×10^9/l ($180\,000$/mm^3).

(*a*) What was the differential diagnosis?
(*b*) What further investigations were required?

Question 6.18

A woman aged 66 years developed sudden back pain. Investigations: X-ray showed crush fracture of L2 vertebrae; serum calcium 2.55 mmol/l (10.2 mg/100 ml); serum phosphate 1.2 mmol/l (3.7 mg/100 ml); serum albumin 40 g/l (4.0 g/100 ml); alkaline phosphatase 135 iu/l (19 King–Armstrong units/l); γ-glutamyl transpepidase 15 iu/l; serum magnesium 0.9 mmol/l (2.2 mg/100 ml); urine calcium 4.47 mmol/day (190 mg/day).

(*a*) Assuming that no cancer was present what was the diagnosis?
(*b*) How should it be confirmed?
(*c*) Name four conditions which may 'cause' this condition.

Question 6.19

A boy aged 3½ years was brought for examination because of short stature. Birth weight 3.5 kg; weight at presentation 13 kg; height 82.5 cm. Examination: no abnormalities noted. Bone age was found to be approximately 18 months.

What further investigations were required to elucidate the diagnosis?

Question 6.20

With some difficulty blood was obtained from a radial artery. The blood gases were Po_2 100 mmHg (13.3 kPa), Pco_2 24 mmHg (3.2 kPa); and pH was 7.48.

What was the diagnosis?

Question 6.21

Plasma sodium 142, potassium 5.0, chloride 104, bicarbonate 25 mmol/l (mEq/l).

(*a*) What is the anion gap from the above figures?
(*b*) What constitutes the gap?
(*c*) Name two conditions in which the gap is increased.

Question 6.22

A previously healthy woman aged 24 years was found to have hypertension, oedema of the ankles and abdominal distension. Investigations: reducing substance present in urine; proteinuria 3–4 g/day; creatinine clearance 78 ml/min; serum urate 0.597 mmol/l (9.2 mg/100 ml). Shortly after these findings the patient suffered a convulsion.

What was the most likely diagnosis?

Question 6.23

A child aged 1 year presented with global retardation and subsequently developed choreo-athetosis and spasticity. He had features of compulsive self-mutilation. By the age of 5 years he had developed an arthropathy. Investigations: blood urea 3.7 mmol/l (22 mg/100 ml); serum urate 0.83 mmol/l (13.9 mg/100 ml); serum calcium 2.5 mmol/l (10.1 mg/ 100 ml); serum phosphate 0.71 mmol/l (2.2 mg/100 ml).

(*a*) What was the diagnosis?
(*b*) What is the cause of this condition?

Question 6.24

A man aged 27 years, height 206 cm with a high, arched palate and hyperextensible finger joints complained of distorted vision.

What urinary constituent should be measured to confirm or refute the diagnosis?

Question 6.25

A man aged 45 years had an intermittent arthropathy for 10 years. He was found to have a Frederickson's Type IV hyperlipoproteinaemia.

(*a*) What is the probable nature of the arthropathy?
(*b*) What are the biochemical features of Type IV hyperlipoproteinaemia?

Question 6.26

Investigations: blood urea 14.0 mmol/l (84 mg/100 ml); plasma sodium 135, potassium 3.0, bicarbonate 32 mmol/l (mEq/l); anion gap of 12.

(*a*) With what condition are the above findings compatible?
(*b*) What would one expect the urine pH to be?

Question 6.27

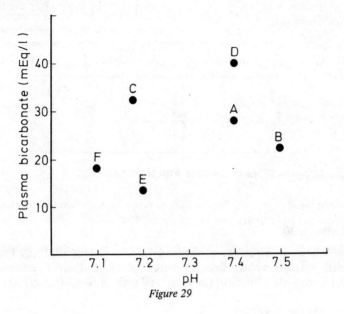

Figure 29

Give diagnoses for points A, B, C, D, E and F on *Figure 29*.

Question 6.28

Investigations: serum calcium 1.97 mmol/l (7.9 mg/100 ml); serum inorganic phosphate 0.8 mmol/l (2.48 mg/100 ml); 25-hydroxyvitamin D_3 (25-OHD$_3$) 25% of standard reference sera.

(a) Suggest two diagnoses.
(b) What symptoms may such a patient have?

Question 6.29

The following venous blood glucose concentrations were found after a 50 g glucose load was given to a woman aged 39 years after she had fasted overnight.

	Glucose	
Time (min)	(mmol/l)	(mg/100 ml)
0	4.3	77
30	6.3	113
60	6.9	124
90	4.9	88
120	4.4	79

Name two conditions compatible with these figures.

Question 6.30

The following results were obtained from a patient who had had a partial gastrectomy two days previously: plasma sodium 75, potassium 2.7, bicarbonate 13 mmol/l (mEq/l); total protein 63 g/l (6.3 g/100 ml).

What was the diagnosis?

Question 6.31

Investigations: blood glucose 10.8 mmol/l (196 mg/100 ml); plasma potassium 6.5 mmol/l (mEq/l); blood urea 4.7 mmol/l (28 mg/100 ml); plasma noradrenaline 805 pg/ml; urine metanephrines 17 μmol/24 h (3.1 mg/day); urinary hydroxymethoxymandelic acid 52 μmol/24 h (10.3 mg/day).

(a) With what diagnosis are the above data compatible?
(b) What one drug could reduce all abnormal concentrations to normal?

Question 6.32

Investigations: plasma sodium 120, potassium 3.6, bicarbonate 27 mmol/l (mEq/l); blood urea 4.7 mmol/l (28 mg/100 ml).

What diagnoses are compatible with the above data?

Question 6.33

A woman aged 35 years was found to have a blood pressure of 165/
105 mmHg. She was treated with diuretics and found to be hypokalaemic.
Further investigation showed a plasma pH of 7.48 and an increased
urinary aldosterone excretion.

(a) Suggest two diagnoses.
(b) Suggest how the differential diagnosis can be resolved.

Question 6.34

A woman aged 29 years had dyspepsia and haematuria. Investigations:
Hb 11.3 g/dl (g/100 ml); MCHC 27 g/dl (g/100 ml) with a hypochromic
microcytic film; blood urea 5.2 mmol/l (31 mg/100 ml); serum calcium
2.95 mmol/l (11.8 mg/100 ml); serum albumin 41 g/l (4.1 g/100 ml);
serum magnesium 1.2 mmol/l (2.9 mg/100 ml); serum phosphate
0.76 mmol/l (2.35 mg/100 ml); alkaline phosphatase 71 iu/l (10 King–
Armstrong units/100 ml); serum urate 0.25 mmol/l (4.2 mg/100 ml);
urine calcium excretion 8.6 mmol/day (345 mg/day); urine culture—
E. coli were covered.

(a) What were the diagnoses?
(b) Name two radiological confirmatory investigations.
(c) Name a biochemical confirmatory test.

Question 6.35

A man aged 71 years with deteriorating severe backache developed
dribbling post-micturition and nocturia. Investigations: Hb 11.5 g/dl
(g/100 ml); ESR 70 mm in the first hour (Westergren); serum calcium
2.3 mmol/l (9.2 mg/100 ml); serum phosphate 1.0 mmol/l (3.1 mg/
100 ml); alkaline phosphatase 206 iu/l (29 King–Armstrong units/
100 ml); total acid phosphatase 10.2 iu/l (5.6 King–Armstrong
units/100 ml).

(a) What were the likely diagnoses?
(b) How may they be confirmed?

Question 6.36

A bottle-fed male baby aged 3 weeks was brought to casualty in a state of collapse with a history of diarrhoea and vomiting for one day. Investigations: Hb 16 g/dl (g/100 ml); PCV 49%; blood urea 10 mmol/l (60 mg/100 ml); plasma sodium 150, potassium 3.5, bicarbonate 14 mmol/l (mEq/l).

(a) What diagnoses would be considered?
(b) What additional investigations should be performed?

Question 6.37

With what conditions are the following data compatible: plasma sodium 144, potassium 2.9, bicarbonate 35 mmol/l (mEq/l); blood urea 5.5 mmol/l (36 mg/100 ml)?

Question 6.38

A woman aged 62 years with a controlled congestive heart failure developed an acutely tender knee joint. Investigations: Hb 12.9 g/dl (g/100 ml); white blood cell count 11.7 × 10^9/l (11 700 mm^3) with 78% neutrophils; blood urea 8.5 mmol/l (51 mg/100 ml); serum urate 0.65 mmol/l (10.8 mg/100 ml); ANF positive 1 in 5.

(a) What was the diagnosis?
(b) How may it be confirmed?
(c) What drug probably caused this condition?

Question 6.39

An infant aged 11 months was admitted as a 'failure to thrive'. He passed large urine volumes and had a normal blood pressure. Investigations: plasma sodium 140, potassium 2.3, bicarbonate 31 mmol/l (mEq/l); blood urea 2.8 mmol/l (18 mg/100 ml); plasma renin activity was very high as was plasma angiotensin II. Urinary aldosterone and prostaglandin levels were supranormal.

(a) What was the diagnosis?
(b) What morphological confirmation could be obtained?
(c) What is the treatment?

Question 6.40

A previously fit 18-year-old man was drowned. Venous blood taken just before death showed: Hb 9.8 g/dl (g/100 ml); PCV 41%; plasma sodium 123, potassium 6.7, chloride 85 mmol/l (mEq/l); serum magnesium 0.82 mmol/l (1.96 mg/100 ml); arterial P_{O_2} 59 mmHg (7.8 kPa); P_{CO_2} 67 mmHg (8.9 kPa); pH 7.26.

(*a*) Did this patient die of inhalation of fresh or sea water?
(*b*) What terminal arrhythmia did he have?

Chapter 7

Haematology

Question 7.1

An ill woman aged 59 years was found to have a serum iron of 10 μmol/l (56 μg/100 ml) in blood sampled at 4.00 pm. Bone marrow showed normal iron stores.

What is the explanation of these findings?

Question 7.2

A woman aged 39 years suffered a hypoplastic anaemia for 3 years which then recovered. Six months later at follow-up the following results were found: Hb 9.5 g/dl (g/100 ml); bilirubin 70 μmol/l (4.1 mg/100 ml); urine contained urobilinogen and haemosiderin; reticulocyte count 12%; red blood cell fragility increased; red blood cell cholinesterase decreased; white blood cell count 2.9 × 10^9/l (2900/mm³); platelets 100 × 10^9/l (100 000/mm³).

(a) What was the diagnosis?
(b) What additional investigations are indicated?
(c) What tests will prove the diagnosis?

Question 7.3

A patient aged 55 years with rheumatoid arthritis was found to have the following: Hb of 9 g/dl (g/100 ml); MCV 59 fl (μm³); MCHC 28 g/dl (g/100 ml); reticulocyte count 4%; serum iron 15 μmol/l (84 μg/100 ml); iron binding capacity 45%.

(a) What was the diagnosis?
(b) What was the likely cause in this patient?
(c) What is the treatment?

Question 7.4

A patient with the following anaemia was treated with oral and subsequently intramuscular iron without improvement: Hb 8.9 g/dl (g/100 ml); MCHC 27 g/dl (g/100 ml); MCV 69 fl (μm³); the blood film was hypochromic.

(*a*) What two diagnoses are possible?
(*b*) What further investigations are needed?

Question 7.5

A boy aged 4 years was pale and lymph nodes were palpable in his neck. Blood count showed a haemoglobin of 9.0 g/dl (g/100 ml); ESR 40 mm in the first hour (Westergren); white blood cell count 50×10^9/l (50 000/mm³) with a differential count of neutrophils 15%, lymphocytes 12%, lymphoblasts 73%.

(*a*) What was the diagnosis?
(*b*) Outline the first steps of management.
(*c*) What is the treatment?
(*d*) What is the prognosis?

Question 7.6

A man aged 64 years had the following blood count: Hb 10 g/dl (g/100 ml); MCV 110 fl (μm³); reticulocyte count 1%; target cells were seen on a blood film. Bone marrow was normoblastic and a serum vitamin B_{12} was 900 ng/l ($\mu\mu$g/ml).

(*a*) What type of anaemia is this?
(*b*) What organ needs investigation? List five necessary investigations

Question 7.7

In a woman aged 68 years with pernicious (Addisonian) anaemia receiving monthly injections of vitamin B_{12} for 11 years, a routine blood count showed Hb 9 g/dl (g/100 ml); MCHC 26 g/dl (g/100 ml); MCV 67 fl (μm³); reticulocyte count 0.6%. The blood film showed microcytes.

What was the probable diagnosis?

Question 7.8

A woman aged 29 years consulted her general practitioner because of chronic fatigue. The Hb was 8.7 g/dl (g/100 ml); MCHC 26 g/dl (g/100 ml); MCV 63 fl (μm^3); reticulocyte count 0.3%; the blood film showed microcytes and hypochromasia. Serum iron 5 μmol/l (28 μg/100 ml) and iron binding capacity 98 μmol/l (498 μg/100 ml).

(a) What was the diagnosis?
(b) Name three common causes in this age group.

Question 7.9

A boy aged 3 years presented with persistent epistaxis. Hb 12.0 g/dl (g/100 ml); white blood cell count 6.7 × 10^9/l (6700/mm^3); platelet count 190 × 10^9/l (190 000/mm^3); bleeding and coagulation times normal; prothrombin time 13 seconds with control 12 seconds; PTT (plasma partial thromboplastin time) 70 seconds, control 34 seconds; PTT with 50% normal plasma 43 seconds.

What was the diagnosis?

Question 7.10

Three days after a haematemesis in a Shipping Director aged 32 years the following blood results were reported: Hb 9.5 g/dl (g/100 ml); PCV 32%; MCHC 30 g/dl (g/100 ml); blood film — microcytes, aniso-cytosis and macrocytosis.

How are these results explained?

Question 7.11

A man aged 60 years who had received ^{32}P for polycythaemia rubra vera 6 years previously, became unwell. Blood examination showed: Hb 9.8 g/dl (g/100 ml); MCHC 30 g/dl (g/100 ml); MCV 94 fl (μm^3); white blood cell count 10 × 10^9/l (10 000/mm^3) with a differential count of neutrophils 53%, lymphocytes 31%, eosinophils 4%, monocytes 7% and myeloblasts 5%.

(a) What was the diagnosis?
(b) What would a bone marrow aspirate show?
(c) What is the prognosis?

Question 7.12

A man of 55 complained of puritis. The haemoglobin was found to be 18.8 g/dl (g/100 ml); PCV 58%; MCV 80 fl (μm^3); white blood cell count 9.3 × 10^9/l (9300/mm^3) with a normal differential count; the blood film showed a few nucleated red cells. Calcium, phosphate and other electrolytes were normal.

(a) What was the diagnosis?
(b) What four tests are necessary to confirm the diagnosis?
(c) List possible treatments.

Question 7.13

A man aged 50 years lost appetite and weight. Blood examination showed: Hb 10.9 g/dl (g/100 ml); PCV 39%; MCHC 30 g/dl (g/100 ml); white blood cell count 12.8 × 10^9/l (12 800/mm^3), with a differential count of neutrophils 64%, lymphocytes 27%, monocytes 3%, myelocytes 2% and metamyelocytes 4%. Scanning of the blood film showed nucleated red blood cells and platelets were frequent in number.

(a) What is this type of blood picture?
(b) How should it be confirmed?
(c) Name five possible underlying conditions.

Question 7.14

A boy aged 10 years developed spontaneous bruising. Many petechiae were present. Investigations: Hb 14.2 g/dl (g/100 ml); white blood cell count 5.5 × 10^9/l (5500/mm^3) with a normal differential; platelets 63 × 10^9/l (63 000/mm^3); the blood film showed that the platelets were large and misshapen.

(a) What was the diagnosis?
(b) What is the treatment?
(c) If the condition became chronic what additional investigation and treatment would be necessary?

Question 7.15

A woman with grey hair and vitiligo became anaemic. The MCV was 120 fl (μm^3) and hypersegmented neutrophils were seen on the blood film.

(a) What was the diagnosis?
(b) Name the three tests to prove the diagnosis.
(c) Suggest two immunological tests that are likely to be positive in this condition.

Question 7.16

In what three conditions may a platelet count of 1000×10^9/l (1 000 000/mm^3) be found?

Question 7.17

A breast-fed male infant aged 3 days oozed blood persistently from the umbilical stump. Investigations: Hb 13.7 g/dl (g/100 ml); PCV 48%; platelets 155 × 10^9/l (155 000/mm^3), white blood cell count 13.5 × 10^9/l (13 500/mm^3), 60% neutrophils, 15% monocytes, 25% lymphocytes; bleeding time 4 minutes; prothrombin time 52 seconds with a control of 15 seconds; fibrinogen concentration 0.14 g/l (140 mg/100 ml).

(a) What was the diagnosis?
(b) What is the treatment?

Question 7.18

A patient had an ileal resection for Crohn's disease. One year later the haemoglobin was found to be 9.2 g/dl (g/100 ml); reticulocyte count 1.3%; MCV 118 fl (μm^3); MCH 39 pg ($\mu\mu$g); platelets 100 × 10^9/l (100 000 mm^3); white blood cell count 1.5 × 10^9/l (1500/mm^3) with a neutropenia; serum vitamin B_{12} 79 ng/l ($\mu\mu$g/ml); serum folate 15 μg/l (μmg/ml); antibodies to gastric parietal cells positive 1 in 128; bone marrow aspirate showed megaloblastic changes. A Schilling test showed low urinary excretion of labelled vitamin B_{12} when the vitamin was given alone and with intrinsic factor.

(a) What was the diagnosis?
(b) How could this be tested easily?

Question 7.19

A man aged 73 years had the following findings: Hb 8.2 g/dl (g/100 ml); blood film — normochromic and hypochromic cells; reticulocyte count 0.7%. Oral iron was given for 6 weeks without increase in the haemoglobulin. Further investigations: faecal occult blood not detected; barium meal and enema normal; serum iron 45 μmol/l (252 μg/100 ml); iron binding capacity 50% saturated; MCHC 30 g/dl (g/100 ml); white blood cell count 4.7 × 10^9/l (4700/mm^3) with a normal differential.

(*a*) What was the probable diagnosis?
(*b*) What would a bone marrow show?

Question 7.20

Name six investigations of a leuco-erythroblastic blood picture.

Figure 7.21

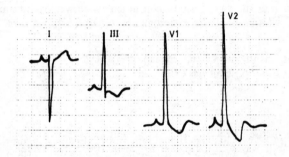

Figure 30

The ECG in *Figure 30* was obtained from a man aged 53 years with a Hb of 20 g/dl (g/100 ml) and a red blood cell count of 7.1 × 10^{12}/l (7.1 × 10^6/mm^3).

(*a*) What does the ECG show?
(*b*) Name two possible associations between the ECG and the haematological findings.

Question 7.22

During investigation of a megaloblastic anaemia 2.0 μg of radioactive vitamin B_{12} were given orally and 1000 μg of non-labelled vitamin B_{12} were given intramuscularly one hour later. Urine was collected for 48 hours and contained 11% of the labelled vitamin B_{12}.

Of what is this diagnostic?

Question 7.23

A man with a known blind loop had the following results: Hb 10.7 g/dl (g/100 ml); reticulocyte count 2.2%; serum iron 12 μmol/l (67 μg/100 ml); iron-binding capacity 78 μmol/l (437 μg/100 ml); serum vitamin B_{12} 80 ng/l ($\mu\mu$g/ml); serum folate 24 μg/l (μmg/ml).

(a) In what range would you expect the MCV to be?
(b) What will a Schilling test show?
(c) Comment upon the serum folate.
(d) How are these findings explained?

Question 7.24

A patient with a megaloblastic marrow was treated with vitamin B_{12} when the Hb was 7.9 g/dl (g/100 ml). There was a 9% reticulocyte count on the 4th day. Despite continued twice weekly intramuscular doses of vitamin B_{12} the haemoglobin failed to rise above 10 g/dl (g/100 ml).

(a) What was the most likely explanation?
(b) What other possibilities exist?

Question 7.25

A boy aged 8 years had a petichial rash and bled from the gums. He had recently suffered from German measles. Investigations: Hb 11.1 g/dl (g/100 ml); white blood cell count 4.5 × 10^9/l (4500/mm^3) with a normal differential count; platelet count 20 × 10^9/l (20 000/mm^3); prothrombin time 18 seconds with a control time of 13 seconds; rubella haemagglutination inhibition (HAI) titre 1 in 28; bone marrow aspirate normal.

(a) Comment upon these figures.
(b) What was the diagnosis?
(c) What other investigations would be useful?
(d) What is the treatment?

Question 7.26

A woman aged 62 years presented with progressive jaundice. Investigations: bilirubin 402 μmol/l (23.5 mg/100 ml); alkaline phosphatase 873 iu/l (123 King–Armstrong Units/100 ml); alanine transaminase (SGPT) 32 iu/l; γ-glutamyl transpepidase 20 iu/l; haemoglobin 11.5 g/dl (g/100 ml); ESR 43 mm in the first hour (Westergren); platelets 275 × 10⁹/l (275 000/mm³); prothrombin time 22 seconds, control 13 seconds; partial thromboplastin time 45 seconds, control 35 seconds; thromboplastin time 13 seconds, control 12 seconds; when normal plasma was added to the patient's plasma the PTT fell to 37 seconds.

(a) What was the overall diagnosis?
(b) What was the cause of the coagulation deficiency?

Question 7.27

Measurements made from cord blood of a second child of an unbooked mother aged 26 years were: Hb 13.0 g/dl (g/100 ml); bilirubin 65 μmol/l (3.8 mg/100 ml); blood group B, Rhesus positive to anti-D.

(a) What was the probable diagnosis?
(b) What is the differential diagnosis?
(c) What further investigations were necessary?

Question 7.28

Which of the following are prognostically significant in a 70 kg man aged 59 years with multiple myeloma and MCV 110 fl (μm³); Hb 12.5 g/dl (g/100 ml); vitamin B₁₂ 750 ng/l (750 μμg/ml); serum albumin 33 g/l (3.3 g/100 ml); serum calcium 2.95 mmol/l (11.8 mg/100 ml); serum urate 0.51 mmol/l (8.7 mg/100 ml); plasma creatinine 305 μmol/l (3.5 mg/100 ml); tumour mass of 10¹² cells/m²; infrequent lytic lesions; λ and κ chains in the urine; IgG concentration 41 g/l (4.1 g/100 ml); IgA 57 g/l (5.7 g/100 ml); urine calcium 44 mmol/day (175 mg/day)?

Question 7.29

Which of the following investigations would help differentiate between myelofibrosis and an adult chronic granulocytic (myeloid) leukaemia?

(*i*)   Red blood cell morphology.
(*ii*)   Serum vitamin B_{12} concentration.
(*iii*) Vitamin B_{12} binding proteins.
(*iv*) Philadelphia chromosome.
(*v*)   Platelet count.
(*vi*) Leucocyte alkaline phosphatase score.
(*vii*) White blood cell count.
(*viii*) Osteosclerosis.

Question 7.30

An English child aged 3 years who had been taken to various Mediterranean and African resorts twice annually presented with epistaxis, weight loss, lymphadenopathy, swollen abdomen and irritability. Investigations: Hb 9.9 g/dl (g/100 ml); MCHC 30 g/dl (g/100 ml); MCV 77 fl (μm^3); platelets 99 $\times$ 10^9/l (99 000/mm^3); white blood cell count 2.9 $\times$ 10^9/l (2900/mm^3); 87% lymphocytes; serum IgG 61.0 g/l (6100 mg/100 ml); Coombs' test positive; bone marrow — normoblastic, no leukaemic changes but clusters of ovoid bodies 2–4 μm in diameter containing two masses of chromatin material were present.

What was the diagnosis?

Question 7.31

An immigrant child aged 7 months was referred because the white blood cell count was found to be 17.0 $\times$ 10^9/l (17 000/mm^3) and leukaemia was feared. Further investigations: platelet count 210 $\times$ 10^9/l (210 000/mm^3); blood film — few myelocytes and myeloblasts, some nucleated red blood cells, marked poikilocytosis and target cells present; MCHC 26 g/dl (g/100 ml); MCV 57 fl (μm^3); reticulocyte count 7%.

(*a*) What was the probable diagnosis?
(*b*) What physical signs were expected?
(*c*) What confirmatory investigation was needed?
(*d*) Name two characteristic X-ray appearances of this condition.

68

Question 7.32

A man aged 24 years presented with right upper abdominal quadrant pain, tenderness and fever. Investigations: urine – bile present; plasma bilirubin 128 μmol/l (7.5 mg/100 ml); alkaline phosphatase 206 iu/l (29 King–Armstrong units/100 ml); alanine transaminase (SGPT) 35 iu/l; Hb 9.9 g/dl (g/100 ml); MCHC 38 g/dl (g/100 ml); MCV 83 fl (μm^3); blood film – red blood cells smaller and darker than normal; Coombs' test negative; reticulocyte count 9.9%.

(*a*) What were the diagnoses?
(*b*) What additional history was necessary?
(*c*) What other physical signs would have been expected?

Question 7.33

A nurse aged 21 years had been febrile and unwell for 12 days when the following investigations became available: bilirubin 85.5 μmol/l (5 mg/100 ml); alanine transaminase (SGPT) 37 iu/l; alkaline phosphatase 106 iu/l (15 King–Armstrong units/100 ml); urine – bile and urobilinogen present; serum IgM 3.1 g/l (310 mg/100 ml); IgA 1.1 g/l (110 mg/100 ml); IgG 2.0 g/l (2000 mg/100 ml); there was a neutropenia and an absolute lymphocytosis; Hb 10.5 g/dl (g/100 ml); reticulocyte count 6%; Coombs' test positive.

(*a*) What was the diagnosis?
(*b*) State two serological confirmatory tests.

Question 7.34

A child aged 4 years presented with listlessness. Investigations: Hb 9.5 g/dl (g/100 ml); blood film – much morphological variation between erythrocytes including cigar-shaped cells and target cells; red blood cell osmotic fragility was decreased; haemoglobin electrophoresis abnormal; sodium metabisulphite test positive; reticulocyte count 7–12%; white blood cell count 15 $\times$ 10^9/l (15 000/mm^3) with a normal differential.

What was the diagnosis?

Question 7.35

A girl aged 14 months suffered a cold and mild diarrhoea and vomiting for 20 hours with a little blood in the stools. On admission she was not dehydrated and there were a few petichiae. Investigations: blood urea 10 mmol/l (60 mg/100 ml); plasma sodium 148, potassium 4.5, bicarbonate 18 mmol (mEq/l); Hb 10.2 g/dl (g/100 ml); platelet count 100×10^9/l (100 000/mm^3).

(a) Comment on the above figures.
(b) What was the diagnosis?
(c) What further tests confirm it?
(d) Predict the clinical course.

Chapter 8
Endocrinology

Question 8.1

A woman aged 27 years had a bitemporal headache and was found to have a diastolic blood pressure of 105 mmHg. Investigations: plasma potassium 3.1 mmol/l (mEq/l); serum cortisol measured at 09.00 hours 990 nmol/l (35.8 µg/100 ml). She was given dexamethasone 8 mg daily. On day 2 serum cortisol was 340 nmol/l (12.3 µg/100 ml) and on day 3 sampled at the same time serum cortisol was 130 nmol/l (4.7 µg/100 ml).

(a) What was the diagnosis?
(b) How may the condition be treated?

Question 8.2

A man aged 51 years developed weakness of his legs. Investigations: serum cortisol at 09.00 hours was 1150 nmol/l (41.5 µg/100 ml) and at 24.00 hours 1090 nmol/l (39.5 µg/100 ml). After 48 hours of dexamethasone 8 mg per day the serum cortisol was 1024 nmol/l (37.1 µg/100 ml) at 09.00 hours.

(a) What is the differential diagnosis?
(b) Give two reasons for the weakness of his legs.

71

Question 8.3

A girl aged 4 years with abnormal facies and on the third percentile for
height and tenth percentile for weight was seen for chronic constipation.
Investigations: Hb 12.8 g/dl (g/100 ml); serum calcium 1.62 mmol/l
(6.48 mg/100 ml); serum phosphate 2.9 mmol/l (8.9 mg/100 ml);
plasma creatinine 44 μmol/l (0.5 mg/100 ml).

(a) What was the diagnosis?
(b) Name two further investigations needed.
(c) Name three of the facial features.

Question 8.4

A female aged 44 years had a T3 binding test of 140% and a plasma
thyroxine of 34.7 nmol/l (2.7 μg/100 ml). Fasting plasma thyroid-
stimulating hormone (TSH) was not detected. Following intravenous
thyrotrophin-releasing hormone (TRH) the plasma TSH was 10 times
above normal control values.

(a) What was the diagnosis?
(b) What else should be considered?

Question 8.5

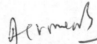

A man aged 29 years presented with visual difficulties, had excessive
sweating and an arthropathy. Investigations: ^{51}Cr EDTA (ethylenediamine
tetra-acetic acid) 144 ml/min; urine calcium excretion 9.9 mmol/day
(394 mg/day) when taking a diet containing less than 500 mg of calcium
daily; serum calcium 2.6 mmol/l (10.4 mg/100 ml); serum phosphate
1.7 mmol/l (5.3 mg/100 ml); alkaline phosphatase 106.5 iu/l (King–
Armstrong units/100 ml). Treatment was given and all abnormal biochemical measurements became normal in 3 months.

(a) What was the diagnosis?
(b) What additional two investigations were essential to make the
diagnosis?

Question 8.6

A man aged 50 years presented with a red face and right heart failure. Urinary assay of a single compound established the diagnosis. Symptomatic improvement followed oral phenoxybenzamine 10 mg three times daily. *CARCINOID*

(*a*) What was the diagnosis?
(*b*) What urinary assay was performed?
(*c*) Name four other features of this condition.

Question 8.7

A woman aged 45 years presented with weight loss, constipation and vomiting. Investigations: calcium 3.05 mmol/l (12.2 mg/100 ml); plasma phosphate 0.6 mmol/l, alkaline phosphatase 135 iu/l (19 King–Armstrong units/100 ml); random TSH 4.7 mU/l (normal range less than 1.0–3.5 mU/l); a Mantoux test negative; white blood cell count 11.7 × 10⁹/l (11 700/mm³), 80% neutrophils, 19% lymphocytes, 1% monocytes. Fasting blood glucose 4.5 mmol/l (81 mg/100 ml).

What was the diagnosis? *?? Hypercalcaemia*

Question 8.8

A patient aged 40 years with proven total anterior pituitary failure was treated with thyroxine and cortisol. After an initial improvement he developed nocturia. At 08.00 hours one morning he weighed 73.2 kg, the urine osmolarity was 330 mmol/l and plasma osmolarity 293 mmol/l. Fluid was withheld for 8 hours, when the measurements were repeated: weight was then 69.7 kg, urine osmolarity 239 mmol/l and plasma osmolarity 301 mmol/l.

(*a*) What do these figures demonstrate?
(*b*) Why did nocturia develop in this man?

Question 8.9

A woman aged 40 years, height 1.75 m, was investigated because of loss of libido and hair together with cold intolerance: serum thyroxine 23 nmol/l (1.8 μg/100 ml); serum TSH 0.2 μg/ml; serum cortisol at 09.00 hours 135 nmol/l (4.9 μg/100 ml); fasting blood glucose 3.4 mmol/l (61 mg/100 ml); plasma ACTH 5 pg/ml; plasma growth hormone fasting 0.8 ng/ml; plasma growth hormone after 1 hour deep sleep 0.5 ng/ml.

(*a*) What was the diagnosis?
(*b*) List six other features of this condition.

Question 8.10

A man aged 39 years with a 4 year history had a heel pad thickness which had increased to 34 mm. Investigations: serum thyroxine 41 nmol/l (3.2 μg/100 ml); T3 uptake 130%; plasma testosterone 3 nmol/l (0.05 μg/ 100 ml); serum cortisol at 09.00 hours 40–105 nmol/l (1.4–3.8 μg/ 100 ml). Fifteen units of soluble insulin and 200 μg TRH were given intravenously. The following results were obtained from blood taken 30 minutes after the intravenous injections: blood glucose 1.9 mmol/l (34 mg/100 ml); growth hormone 0.9 mU/l; plasma cortisol 205 nmol/l (7.4 ng/ml); TSH 5 mU/l.

What were the diagnoses?

Question 8.11

A woman aged 59 years complained of increasing tiredness for 6 months. Investigations: plasma sodium 130, potassium 6.1, chloride 96, bicarbonate 23 mmol/l (mEq/l); blood urea 6 mmol/l (36 mg/100 ml).

(*a*) What was the probable diagnosis?
(*b*) Name one test which will support or refute the diagnosis.

Question 8.12

In a patient suspected of having either Cushing's syndrome or atopic ACTH production which of the following aid in the differential diagnosis: blood glucose; cortisol production rate studies; plasma ACTH of 280 pg/ml; the urinary changes in 17-hydroxycorticosteroid (17-OHCS) after metyrapone; changes in urinary excretion of 17-OHCS after 8 mg of dextramethazone for 48 hours?

Question 8.13

Name three conditions in which the basal metabolic rate (BMR) is raised.

Question 8.14

A patient with established hyperthyroidism was treated with carbimazole 30 mg daily for 4 months. Investigations at this time: serum thyroxine 85 nmol/l (6.6 μg/100 ml); protein bound iodine (PBI) 485 nmol/l (6.1 μg/100 ml). Seventy-two hours after withdrawing carbimazole 58% of a tracer dose of I^{131} was taken up by the thyroid gland.

What discrepancy is there in these results and how is it explained?

Question 8.15

With what diagnoses are the following laboratory investigations compatible: serum cholesterol 4 mmol/l (155 mg/100 ml); PBI 1000 nmol/l (12.7 μg/100 ml); T4 (serum thyroxine) 180 nmol/l (14.7 μg/100 ml); I^{131} uptake at 24 hours 53%; serum T3 uptake test 20% less than usual laboratory range?

What further information would be needed for a more precise diagnosis?

Question 8.16

A widow aged 70 years sought advice for tingling and numbness in the fingers. She was also constipated and moderately deaf. All features were of 6 months duration. Investigations revealed pernicious anaemia and after 6 months of treatment with vitamin B_{12} the anaemia was corrected but her original symptoms were unchanged.

(a) What was the diagnosis?
(b) How is it related to her anaemia?
(c) List 15 further features of this condition.

Question 8.17

The following blood glucose concentrations were obtained from venous blood taken from a patient who had been given a 50 g glucose load after an overnight fast:

Time (min)	Glucose (mmol/l)	(mg/100 ml)
0	4.5	81
30	11.2	202
60	5.4	97
90	3.3	60
120	4.1	74

(*a*) What type of curve was this?
(*b*) Mention three conditions in which it may be found.

Question 8.18

A man aged 49 years had a haemoptysis and was found to have an abnormal chest X-ray. Plasma potassium 2.9, bicarbonate 33 mmol/l (mEq/l); glycosuria was found.

(*a*) What was the diagnosis?
(*b*) What is the prognosis?

Question 8.19

The following were found in a baby 1 week old with intermediate genitalia: buccal smear chromatin positive; karyotype 46 XX; urinary ketosteroids 185 μmol/24 h (0.5 mg/24 h).

(*a*) Comment upon the results.
(*b*) What is the differential diagnosis of intermediate genitalia?
(*c*) What further investigations may be indicated?

Question 8.20

A talkative male aged 32 years presented with loss of libido of 2 years duration. His weight had increased, gynaeocomastia and soft testes were present. Investigations: ESR 24 mm in the first hour (Westergren); plasma testosterone 6.5 nmol/l; plasma prolactin 247 μg/l. Thyroid-releasing factor (TRF) did not increase the prolactin concentration. *Hyperolactinaemia*

(a) What was the differential diagnosis?
(b) What additional investigations were needed?

Question 8.21

Three days after removal of a chronically rejected transplant kidney, blood taken at 08.00 hours had a serum cortisol concentration of 140 nmol/l (5.0 μg/100 ml). A dose of synthetic ACTH was given intramuscularly. Thirty minutes later the serum cortisol was 395 nmol/l (14.3 μg/100 ml).

What was the diagnosis?

Question 8.22

A healthy insulin-dependent diabetic aged 23 years attended her doctor because of recent evening fainting attacks. Testing of urine at the time of these episodes showed ¾–1% glycosuria. She had not recently changed her dose of insulin. Blood glucose concentrations at 08.00, 12.00, 16.00 and 20.00 hours the following day were 10.3 (185), 13.2 (237), 6.8 (123) and 4.7 (85) mmol/l (mg/100 ml) respectively.

(a) What was the diagnosis?
(b) What underlying condition was present? *Pregnancy*

Chapter 9
Immunology

Question 9.1

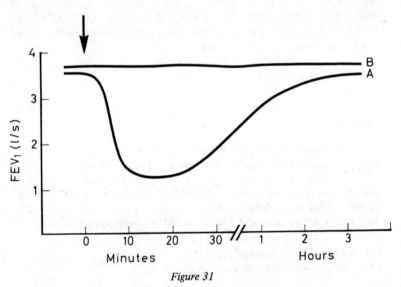

Figure 31

An endobronchial chalange by an antigen was given at zero time. The FEV$_1$ was measured repeatedly as shown in *Figure 31* (Trace A). The following day the patient received a drug (arrow) 2 minutes before an identical chalange (Trace B).

(*a*) What was the diagnosis?
(*b*) What is the mediation of this reaction?
(*c*) What drug was given before the second experiment?

78

Question 9.2

A boy aged 4 years suffered from eczema and had a history of infections and bruising. Investigations: Hb 8.5 g/dl (g/100 ml); platelet count $70 \times 10^9/l$ (70 000/mm^3); serum IgM 0.3 g/l (300 mg/100 ml); IgA 3.8 g/l (3800 mg/100 ml); IgG 4.7 g/l (4700 mg/100 ml); T-cell count 172 spontaneous sheep red blood cell rosettes/mm^3; B-cell count 343/mm^3.

(a) What was the diagnosis?
(b) What is the mode of inheritance?
(c) What pathological abnormalities were present?
(d) What forms of treatment are available?

Question 9.3

(a) Which disease in the following list is unlikely to be associated with other diseases in the list?

  Systemic lupus erythematosus
  Discoid lupus erythematosus
  Pernicious anaemia
  Sclerodermia
  Rheumatoid arthritis

(b) Why?

Question 9.4

(a) Can a patient who is blood group O receive a kidney from potential donors of blood groups A or B?
(b) Can a patient who has a genotype AB receive a donor kidney from:

  (i) a patient with genotype OO?
  (ii) a patient of blood group B?

Question 9.5

A patient aged 67 years with seropositive rheumatoid arthritis developed weakness of dorsiflexion of the right foot, the ankle of which was normal.

(a) What is seropositivity in this context?
(b) How is it mediated?
(c) Name one clinical test which would help clarify the weakness of dorsiflexion.

Question 9.6

A patient with an auto-immune arthropathy developed pericardial and pleural effusions: albumin content 17 g/l (1.7 g/100 ml); glucose concentration 2.1 mmol/l (38 mg/100 ml); C3 10% of normal reference serum; C4 8% of normal reference serum; cells $1.1 \times 10^9/l$ (1100/mm^3), 84% lymphocytes, 12% eosinophils, 4% polymorphs. In addition elongated multinucleate cells were found in the pleural fluid.

(a) What was the diagnosis?
(b) What serum factor would establish the diagnosis?
(c) What type of effusions are these?
(d) What is the differential diagnosis of the pleural effusion?

Question 9.7

A woman aged 26 years, having had active Still's disease since the age of 10, developed increased ankle oedema. Investigations: ESR 60 mm in the first hour (Westergren); Hb 10.7 g/dl (g/100 ml); MCHC 30 g/dl (g/100 ml); MCH 31 pg ($\mu\mu$g); 24 hour urine protein excretion 13.7 g; creatinine clearance 39 ml/min; plasma albumin 27 g/l (2.7 g/100 ml); urine was found to contain free λ and κ chains; serum immunoglobulins within normal range; rheumatoid factor absent; IVP normal gross anatomy of urinary tract.

(a) What was the main functional renal diagnosis?
(b) Suggest two likely causes.
(c) Suggest two further investigations.

Question 9.8

A woman aged 76 years who had morning stiffness with pectoral and pelvic girdle pain for 9 months suddenly developed severe right temporal pain and noted rapid deterioration of vision in the right eye. The ESR was 89 mm in the first hour (Westergren).

(a) What was the diagnosis?
(b) How may the diagnosis be confirmed?
(c) What is the treatment?
(d) When should treatment be started?

Question 9.9

A child aged 3 months who had been treated for neonatal hypoparathyroidism developed recurrent viral and *Candida* infections. Investigations: immunoglobulin concentrations normal for age; peripheral white blood cell count $3.8 \times 10^9/l$ ($3800/mm^3$), differential count polymorphs 89%, monocytes 1%, lymphocytes 10%. The majority of lymphocytes present bound fluorescent antigen. No spontaneous rosettes formed with sheep red blood cells. It was not possible to induce dinitrochlorobenzene skin sensitization.

(*a*) What was the diagnosis?
(*b*) What will a lymph node biopsy show?
(*c*) What is the treatment?

Question 9.10

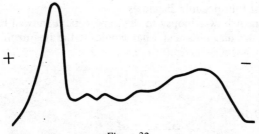

Figure 32

The above electrophoretic strip (*Figure 32*) was obtained from a patient with chronic disease.

(*a*) What abnormal features are shown?
(*b*) Suggest two diagnoses.

Question 9.11

(*a*) On which chromosome are the HLA loci found?
(*b*) How many subloci are there?
(*c*) Name three diseases which appear to have an association with possession of HLA 8.

Question 9.12

A woman aged 23 years presented with a 6 month history of arthropathy, adenopathy, Raynaud's phenomenon and dyspnoea. Investigations: ESR 69 mm in the first hour (Westergren); ANF positive 1:1024 with a speckled nuclear pattern on immunofluorescence; serum gamma globulin 70 g/l (7.0 g/100 ml); DNA binding less than 10%; CH50 97%. A high titre of antibody to ribonuclear protein was demonstrated.

What was the diagnosis?

Question 9.13

During investigation of a rash, a biopsy from an uninvolved area of skin was taken. Immunofluorescence demonstrated the presence of immuno-globulins and C3.

(a) Suggest four possible diagnoses.
(b) If a small bowel biopsy in the same patient showed blunted villi, what was the diagnosis and what would be the treatment of the skin disease?

Question 9.14

With what diseases are the following data compatible: faecal fat excretion 149 mmol (42 g) over a 3 day period; bromsulphathalein retention 19% at 45 minutes; creatinine clearance 40 ml/min.

Question 9.15

A patient with a proven immune complex nephritis developed increased proteinuria. Complement measurements (expressed as a percentage of normal) showed the following: CH50 47%; C4 62%; C3 40%.

Do these measurements indicate:

(i)   classical pathway activation, or
(ii) alternative pathway activation?

Question 9.16

Which of the following investigations would be of value in a possible case of Bruton's syndrome in a boy aged 7 months who had suffered recurrent ear, throat and chest infections: peripheral white blood cell count; bone marrow aspiration; HLA typing; differential B- and T-cell counts; measurements of phagocytosis of *Candida albicans* spores; estimation of lymphokines function; skin testing for dinitrochlorobenzene sensitivity?

Question 9.17

During the investigation of a patient with an MCV of 115 fl (μm^3) fluorescent studies upon material obtained at a jejunal biopsy showed a predominance of IgM containing plasma cells. Serum IgM was 2.5 g/l (250 mg/100 ml) and IgA was not demonstrated by radial immunodiffusion assay.

(a) What was the probable diagnosis?
(b) Explain the findings.
(c) What HLA antigen would you expect this patient to possess?

Question 9.18

A boy aged 3 years with severe combined immune deficiency received an ABO and HLA identical marrow transplant from a female donor. Female polymorphonuclear cells were seen in the peripheral blood 10 days after the transplant but at 18 days the boy developed diarrhoea with a macular eruption of the trunk and then face and hands.

(a) Assuming these signs and symptoms were not related to infection what was the diagnosis?
(b) Name two conditions which are necessary for this reaction to develop.

Question 9.19

A man aged 71 years was admitted because of deteriorating consciousness. He was found to have hepatosplenomegaly, lymphadenopathy and a retinopathy. Investigations: Hb 9.2 g/dl (g/100 ml); MCHC 30 g/dl (g/100 ml); MCV 79 fl (μm^3); MCH 31 pg ($\mu\mu g$); white cell count 4.1 × 10^9/l (4100/mm³), differential count normal; ESR 67 mm in the first hour; prothrombin time 17 seconds, control 12 seconds; partial thromboplastin time 44 seconds, control 35 seconds; platelets 125 × 10^9/l (125 000/mm³); cryoglobulins present; blood viscosity 2.5 × greater than control serum. There was no Bence-Jones proteinuria.

(*a*) What was the probable diagnosis?
(*b*) How may this be confirmed?
(*c*) What retinopathy would one expect to see?
(*d*) What is the treatment?

Question 9.20

A patient received an intradermal dose of antigen to which he had previously been exposed. A reaction began at 6 hours and subsided by 20 hours.

Is this a Type I, II, III or IV reaction and what is the mediation?

Question 9.21

A woman aged 33 years with Raynaud's phenomenon of 5 years' duration reported matutinal finger stiffness and dysphagia. Investigations: ESR 71 mm in the first hour (Westergren); Hb 11.9 g/dl (g/100 ml); reticulocyte count 1.3%; ANF positive 1 in 50; cryoglobulins not detected; rheumatoid factor positive 1 in 2; DNA binding 18%.

What was the diagnosis?

Chapter 10
Pharmacology

Question 10.1

Which of the following drugs could be causal of the following biochemical and haematological measurements?

colchicine	serum urate 119 μmol/l (2 mg/100 ml)
azathioprine	serum urea 33.3 mmol/l (200 mg/100 ml)
cephaloridine	plasma creatinine 380 μmol/l (4.3 mg/100 ml)
methysergide	serum potassium 3.8 mmol/l (mEq/l)
bumetanide	bilirubin 34 μmol/l (2.0 mg/100 ml)
aspirin	proteinuria 8 g/day
digoxin	haemoglobin 11.1 g/dl (g/100 ml)
gentamicin	MCV 109 fl (μm^3)
trimethadione	platelets 58 × 10^9/l (58 000/mm^3)
phenylbutazone	

Question 10.2

A man aged 77 years had progressive hip joint discomfort for 2 years. Investigations: Hb 12.9 g/dl (g/100 ml); white blood cell count 4.9 × 10^9/l (4900/mm^3) with a normal differential; ESR 30 mm in the first hour (Westergren); serum calcium 2.6 mmol/l (10.4 mg/100 ml); serum phosphate 1.4 mmol/l (4.3 mg/100 ml); serum albumin 37 g/l (3.7 g/100 ml); alkaline phosphatase 212 iu/l (30 King–Armstrong units/100 ml); serum urate 0.46 mmol/l (7.7 mg/100 ml); urine calcium 8.3 mmol/24 hours (332 mg/24 hours); urine hydroxyproline excretion raised.

(*a*) What was the diagnosis?
(*b*) What is the explanation of the abnormal findings?
(*c*) What drugs are available to treat this condition?

Question 10.3

A Turkish woman aged 35 years presented with dependent oedema. The past history included multiple attacks of abdominal pain and an arthropathy. Investigations: creatinine clearance 49 ml/min; serum urate 0.38 mmol/l (6.4 mg/100 ml); serum albumin 27 g/l (2.7 g/100 ml); serum cholesterol 14.5 mmol/l (561 mg/100 ml).

(a) What was the immediate diagnosis?
(b) What was the overall diagnosis?
(c) What treatment should be given for (a) and (b)?

Question 10.4

A man aged 45 years with treated moderate hypertension left for a business trip. About 36 hours after leaving home he attended a casualty department complaining of headache, agitation, sweating and palpitations. The blood pressure was 220/145 mmHg. He was admitted and investigation showed a urinary catecholamine excretion of 15 μmol/24 hours (274 mg/24 hours).

(a) What was the differential diagnosis?
(b) What hypotensive agent had he left at home?
(c) What is the treatment of this condition and with what drug?

Question 10.5

A hypertensive West Indian receiving diazoxide therapy was admitted semicomatose. Investigations: blood glucose 70 mmol/l (1260 mg/100 ml); serum sodium 155 mmol/l (mEq/l); serum potassium 3.2 mmol/l (mEq/l); serum urea 8.4 mmol/l (55 mg/100 ml). There was no ketonuria.

(a) What was the diagnosis?
(b) What was the plasma osmolarity?
(c) Outline the treatment.

Question 10.6

A man with an acute exacerbation of chronic bronchitis was admitted to hospital and received treatment. After 6 hours he was found to have deteriorated. Arterial blood findings were: Po_2 108 mmHg (14.4 kPa); Pco_2 141 mmHg (18.8 kPa); pH 7.21.

(a) What was the diagnosis?
(b) What error in treatment had been made?
(c) What physical signs are likely to be present?
(d) Outline further treatment.

Question 10.7

A patient with a GFR of 5 ml/min developed bone pain. Serum calcium 2.1 mmol/l (8.3 mg/100 ml); phosphate 3.3 mmol/l (10.3 mg/100 ml); alkaline phosphatase 270 iu/l (35 King–Armstrong units/100 ml). He was subsequently treated with vitamin D in a dose of 100 000 units orally daily. He was seen 6 months later. Investigations: serum calcium 3.55 mmol/l (14.2 mg/100 ml); serum phosphate 2.96 mmol/l (9.2 mg/ 100 ml); alkaline phosphatase 135 iu/l (19 King–Armstrong units/ 100 ml).

(a) What was the original diagnosis?
(b) What was the subsequent diagnosis?
(c) Comment upon management.
(d) What complications may be found?

Question 10.8

A girl aged 17 years with stable renal failure attended her doctor for facial 'spots'. Tablets were prescribed. Ten days later she required hospital admission because of nausea and vomiting. Investigations: Hb 17.5 g/dl (g/100 ml); white blood cell count 17.5×10^9/l (17 500/ mm^3); blood urea 64.8 mmol/l (428 mg/100 ml); urine volume 190 ml in 6 hours; urine osmolarity 305 mmol/l.

(a) What was the diagnosis?
(b) Outline three steps in immediate management.
(c) What drug had she probably been given?

Question 10.9

Four days after a suicide attempt with a single compound the following investigations were available: Hb 12.0 g/dl (g/100 ml); white blood cell count 17.5×10^9/l (17 500 mm^3) with 89% neutrophils; serum phosphate 2.3 mmol/l (7.1 mg/100 ml); serum calcium 2.5 mmol/l (10 mg/100 ml); blood urea 17.2 mmol/l (103 mg/100 ml); arterial pH 7.23; plasma bilirubin 123 μmol/l (7.2 mg/100 ml); alanine transaminase (SGPT) 392 iu/l; prothrombin time 21 seconds, control 14 seconds; alkaline phosphatase 78 iu/l (11 King–Armstrong units/ 100 ml).

Name two compounds that this patient could have taken.

Question 10.10

A child aged 5 years was admitted in status asthmaticus and given intravenous bronchodilators and steroids. The figures below are serial blood gas analyses.

Time (h)	PO_2 (mmHg)	(kPa)	PCO_2 (mmHg)	(kPa)	Bicarbonate (mmol/l)	pH
0	82	10.9	51	6.8	19	7.25
3	108	14.4	102	13.6	22	7.13
5	266	35.5	194	25.9	20.6	6.97
7	225	30.0	62	8.3	25.7	7.32
9	170	22.6	71	9.5	22.5	7.42
14	101	13.5	45	6.0	28	7.43

(*a*) What happened between admission and the 5th hour?
(*b*) What signs would be expected at 5 hours after admission?
(*c*) What was done between the 5th and 7th hours after admission and subsequently up to 14 hours?

Question 10.11

A Caucasian woman of 19 years was found to have a blood pressure of 180/125 mmHg. IVP normal; peripheral venous renin 3490 pg ml^{-1} h^{-1}; blood urea 12 mmol/l (72 mg/100 ml); GFR 48 ml/min; urine microscopy no abnormality; proteinuria 1.9 g/day.

(*a*) What was the diagnosis?

She was successfully treated with oral diazoxide and frusemide. One week later the peripheral venous renin was found to have approximately doubled in concentration and the GFR had fallen to 33 ml/min.

(*b*) Comment upon the increase in the renin and the fall in GFR.
(*c*) Comment upon the drug treatment.

Question 10.12

A woman aged 68 years with atrial fibrillation had been taking 0.25 mg digoxin daily for 9 years. At follow-up she reported anorexia, nausea and vomiting. Her pulse was 97 per minute. Investigations: blood urea 6.8 mmol/l (41 mg/100 ml); plasma creatinine 90 μmol/l (1.0 mg/100 ml); serum potassium 4.7 mmol/l (mEq/l); plasma digoxin 6 hours after the last dose 2.7 ng/ml.

(*a*) What was the diagnosis?
(*b*) What apparent discrepancy is there in the above figures?

Question 10.13

A girl aged 19 years was admitted after a determined suicide attempt with a single drug. Initial blood gases were: Po_2 103 mmHg (13.7 kPa); Pco_2 29 mmHg (3.8 kPa); pH 7.48.

(a) What is this biochemical state called?
(b) What drug had the woman taken?
(c) What acid—base changes may occur later?

Question 10.14

A patient with Frederickson's Type IV hyperlipidaemia was treated with clofibrate and cholestyramine. He developed a venous thrombosis of the right calf and was given intravenous heparin for 48 hours followed by warfarin. On the 3rd day a severe gastrointestinal haemorrhage occurred.

Why?

Question 10.15

From a patient aged 47 years with severe psoriasis the following measurements were made: Hb 10.2 g/dl (g/100 ml); ESR 27 mm in the first hour; white blood cell count 2.2 × 10^9/l (2200/mm^3) with a normal differential count; MCV 117 fl (μm^3), MCHC 32 g/dl (g/100 ml); reticulocyte count 1%; serum B12 540 ng/l ($\mu\mu$g/ml).

(a) How is the anaemia explained?
(b) How is it treated?

Question 10.16

A child aged 4 years was brought to a casualty department unconscious. Temperature 38.2°C. Investigations: CSF clear; white blood cells 3/mm^3; protein 0.5 g/l (50 mg/100 ml); glucose 3.3 mmol/l (60 mg/100 ml); blood urea 9 mmol/l (54 mg/100 ml); plasma sodium 140 mmol/l (mEq/l); plasma bicarbonate 17 mmol/l (mEq/l).

(a) Comment on the figures.
(b) Suggest possible diagnoses and further investigations.

Question 10.17

A man aged 28 years, known for 2 years to have familial hyper-cholesterolaemia and severe hypertriglyceridaemia, developed acute right upper quadrant abdominal pain and tenderness. Investigations: bilirubin 97.5 μmol/l (5.7 mg/100 ml); serum alkaline phosphatase 220 iu/l (31 King–Armstrong units/100 ml); alanine transaminase (SGPT) 137 iu/l; urine contained bile; fasting cholesterol 8.0 mmol/l (310 mg/100 ml); fasting triglycerides 1.9 mmol/l (173 mg/100 ml).

(*a*) What was the diagnosis?
(*b*) What was the probable cause?

Question 10.18

After 2 years of continuous drug therapy a woman aged 27 years sought advice regarding constipation. Investigations: serum calcium 2.79 mmol/l (11.2 mg/100 ml); serum magnesium 1.1 mmol/l (2.6 mg/100 ml); ESR 17 mm in the first hour (Westergren); serum thyroxine 50 mmol/l (3.9 μg/100 ml); T3 uptake 129%.

(*a*) What drug had this patient been taking?
(*b*) Name two other side-effects.

Question 10.19

A severe epileptic aged 30 years gradually developed backache. Investigations: blood urea 3.9 mmol/l (25.7 mg/100 ml); serum albumin 40 g/l (4.0 g/100 ml); serum calcium 2.1 mmol/l (8.4 mg/100 ml); serum inorganic phosphate 0.9 mmol/l (2.8 mg/100 ml); plasma alkaline phosphatase 177 iu/l (25 King–Armstrong units/100 ml); plasma 25-OHD$_3$ 43% of standard reference sera.

(*a*) What was the diagnosis?
(*b*) Why had it occurred?
(*c*) What is the pathogenesis?

Question 10.20

(*a*) What group of drugs may:

    (*i*) decrease urinary urate;
    (*ii*) increase urinary magnesium;
    (*iii*) reduce urinary calcium;
    (*iv*) increase urinary iodide?

(*b*) What metabolic diseases may be associated with this group of drugs?
(*c*) In what condition is one of these properties of therapeutic value?

Question 10.21

A child aged 3 years received phenytoin and phenobarbitone because of epilepsy. The phenytoin level was 2 mg/l and the phenobarbitone level was 4.5 mg/l.

Comment on these figures.

Question 10.22

A man receiving treatment for carcinoma of the prostate developed gynaecomastia and peripheral oedema.

(*a*) What drug did he receive?
(*b*) If he considered gynaecomastia unacceptable what alternative therapy may be offered?

Question 10.23

A man aged 25 years was treated with lithium carbonate for a manic depressive neurosis for 18 months. For the latter 5 months of treatment nocturia was reported. Investigations: urine sterile; blood urea 4.5 mmol/l (22 mg/100 ml); serum electrolytes normal; overnight urine osmolarity 425 mmol/l; plasma lithium concentration 0.9–1.3 mmol/l.

(*a*) What biochemical abnormalities were present?
(*b*) Explain the nocturia.

Question 10.24

In an adult man with a constant plasma creatinine of 256 µmol/l
(2.9 mg/100 ml) which of the following drugs should be avoided:
propranolol, nitrazepam, demethylchlortetracycline, clofibrate, quinal-
barbitone, digoxin, metoclopramide, cephaloridine, ampicillin, spironolactone, nitrofurantoin, co-trimoxazole, sotalol, acebutolol?

Question 10.25

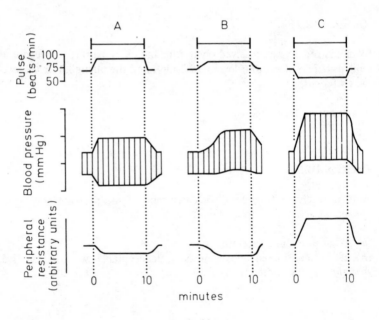

Figure 33

Figure 33 shows pulse, blood pressure and peripheral resistance changes
recorded from a cat under pentobarbitone anaesthesia when three
pharmacological doses of naturally occurring substances were infused
between minutes 0 and 10.

What were substances A, B and C?

Question 10.26

A woman aged 25 years was found to have a blood pressure of 155/110. Investigations: blood urea 4.0 mmol/l (24 mg/100 ml); plasma potassium 3.0, sodium 140, bicarbonate 27 mmol/l (mEq/l); plasma aldosterone 155 pmol/l. She was treated with spironolactone 300 mg daily and in 18 days the blood pressure was 135/90 mmHg.

What was the diagnosis?

Question 10.27

Which of the following combinations of drugs given orally are best avoided: tetracycline and ferrous sulphate; cholestyramine and phenyl-butazone; phenobarbitone and griseofulvin; tetracycline and aluminium hydroxide; para-aminosalicylic acid (PAS) and rifampicin?

Question 10.28

Twenty-four mice were infected with a β-lactamase-producing strain of *Staphalococcus aureus*. They were then treated with a new cephalosporin to determine its *in vivo* effect. A control group of 24 mice received saline injections only. Twenty-one of the treated group survived and all of the control group died.

Which of the following statistical procedures is appropriate for analysis of the results: the binomial distribution; student's t-test, the chi squared (χ^2) test or the method of least squares?

Question 10.29

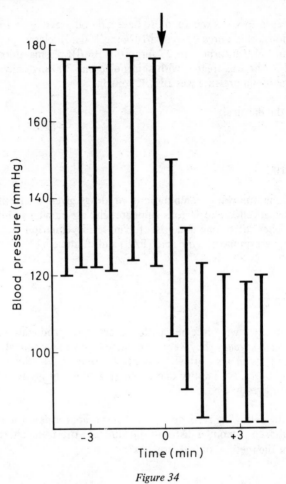

Figure 34

Figure 34 shows a series of blood pressure measurements taken before and after an intravenous drug. The plasma renin before the injection (arrow) was 7800 pg ml⁻¹ h⁻¹.

(*a*) Name five drugs which might have been used.
(*b*) Does knowledge of the plasma renin concentration help in selection of a suitable hypotensive drug from *Figure 34*?
(*c*) Could such a depressor response be diagnostic?

94

Question 10.30

What action is common to all the following drugs: phenylbutazone, carbimazole, PAS, methylthiouracil and lithium?

Question 10.31

An elderly woman with established cirrhosis and portosystemic encephalopathy deteriorated cerebrally despite a low protein diet and neomycin 2 g daily. The dose of neomycin was trebled with improvement in cerebral function but 3 months later the patient developed diarrhoea. Investigations: Hb 10.2 g/dl (g/100 ml); MCV 115 fl (μm^3); white blood cell count 4.5 x 10^9/l (4500/mm^3); alanine transaminase (SGPT) 65 iu/l; serum alkaline phosphatase 248 iu/l (35 King–Armstrong units/100 ml); serum albumin 39 g/l (3.9 g/100 ml); xylose excretion 13% excreted in 7 hours; faecal fat 49.3 mmol/day (14 g/day).

What are the probable diagnoses?

Chapter 11
Answers and Discussion

CARDIOLOGY

Answer 1.1

This child had an atrial septal defect (ASD) with a left-to-right shunt. There was a step up in oxygen saturation in the right atrium when oxygen saturation is usually about 65–70% in this chamber. Because oxygenated blood was gaining access to the right heart oxygen saturation in the right ventricle and pulmonary artery were much higher than usual.

Answer 1.2

The pulmonary arterial pressure was greater than the systemic arterial pressure. There was a high right ventricular systolic pressure but no increased arterial oxygen saturation in that chamber. There was therefore a ventricular septal defect (VSD) with a balanced shunt and pulmonary hypertension – the Eisenmenger syndrome.

Answer 1.3

(a) This child had a VSD as shown by the step up in oxygenation at right ventricular level.
(b) The physical sign is a pansystolic murmur heard at the left sternal edge in the third and fourth intercostal space with or without a systolic thrill.

96

Answer 1.4

This child had an ASD and pulmonary stenosis. The ASD was diagnosed by the step up in oxygen saturation in the right atrium due to a left-to-right shunt. (The further step up in oxygenation in the right ventricle is simply a measure of further mixing of the oxygenated blood from the left heart.) The pulmonary stenosis is shown by the high right ventricular pressure and normal pulmonary artery pressure. The systolic gradient was 41 mmHg which is well into the pathological range. Usually a pulmonary valve gradient is not regarded as significant unless it is more than 20 mmHg as there is a Venturi effect across the valve, giving rise to a small gradient.

Answer 1.5

(*a*) This man had aortic stenosis. There was modest elevation of the right heart pressures and a marked systolic gradient of 68 mmHg across the aortic valve.
(*b*) The treatment is aortic valvular replacement.

Answer 1.6

There was a sharp drop in pressure somewhere in the aorta. The most common cause is coarctation. However this patient had hypercalcaemia and abnormal facies which are associated with supravalvular aortic stenosis. This was the diagnosis in this child.

Answer 1.7

There was a step up in the oxygen saturation in the right ventricle; this was due to a left-to-right shunt via a VSD.

Answer 1.8

(*i*) This child was a male Mongol.
(*ii*) There was a step up in oxygen saturation at atrial level, indicating an ASD which was of the ostium primum type since this lesion is frequently found in Mongols. If all the figures were obtained via a right heart catheter the child would have an endocardial cushion defect since this lesion allows a catheter via the inferior vena cava (IVC) to be manipulated into all the heart chambers.

Answer 1.9

(*a*) The data indicate pulmonary stenosis (high right ventricular pressure and low pulmonary artery pressure) and a VSD with a right-to-left shunt. These are two features of Fallot's tetralogy; the other two components — right ventricular hypertrophy and an over-riding aorta — are demonstrated by ECG and angiography.

(*b*) The postero-anterior (PA) chest X-ray showed:

(*i*) a small pulmonary artery due to low pulmonary artery pressure;
(*ii*) a 'boot-shaped' heart due to right ventricular hypertrophy;
(*iii*) oligaemic lung fields.

Answer 1.10

(*a*) The pulmonary artery wedge pressure was raised which implies raised left atrial pressure. The left ventricular pressures are normal. The diagnosis was therefore pure mitral stenosis.

(*b*) The chest X-ray may show an enlarged left atrium and a small left ventricle. The pulmonary artery may be prominent.

Answer 1.11

(*a*) This child had pure pulmonary stenosis as shown by the pressure gradient between the right ventricle and the pulmonary artery. There was no shunt as there was no step up in oxygen saturation in the right side of the heart.

(*b*) The chest X-ray may show an enlarged main pulmonary artery due to poststenotic dilatation.

Answer 1.12

The pressures indicate mitral incompetence and mitral stenosis. The right heart pressures were raised as was the pulmonary artery wedge pressure. In health, left atrial pressure is equal to the left ventricular end diastolic pressure and also the pulmonary artery wedge pressure. In this patient the gradient across the mitral valve was 16 mmHg (25–9). In an adult a gradient of more than 5 mmHg is usually taken to be clinically significant.

Answer 1.13

(*a*) This patient could also have had diabetes, polyarteritis nodosa or perhaps leukaemia.

(*b*) Untreated diabetics usually have a fasting blood sugar above 8.5 mmol/l (150 mg/100 ml) but if doubt remained a GTT would clarify the diagnosis. Polyarteritis nodosa is often associated with a raised ESR, lung changes and sometimes an eosinophilia. If proteinuria were present a renal biopsy is an easy way to make the diagnosis. Acute leukaemia causing retinal haemorrhages would be associated with thrombocytopaenia and often anaemia. A bone marrow aspirate would be essential.

Answer 1.14

(*a*) A long systolic murmur following a myocardial infarction very probably represents the development of mitral incompetence or a VSD. Either abnormality may be complicated by the development of subacute bacterial endocarditis and this is associated with fever, anaemia, leucocytosis and haematuria.

(*b*) Six blood cultures should be taken in the 24 hours following the presumed diagnosis. *Staphylococcus aureus* is a common pathogen in subacute bacterial endocarditis (SBE) and penicillin treatment should be begun as soon as the cultures have been taken. Echocardiography will differentiate between mitral incompetence and a VSD. After control of the infection left ventricular angiography might well be necessary before surgical repair of the mechanical defect. Surgery may be needed early in the clinical course to excise infected tissue, to patch the VSD or replace the mitral valve.

Answer 1.15

(*a*) This man had a postinfarction ventricular aneurysm as shown by the persistent ST elevation over the left ventricular leads and the bulge on the lateral border of the enlarged heart. This condition is usually associated with total occlusion of the anterior descending branch of the left coronary artery.

(*b*) The essential investigations are left ventricular angiography with coronary arteriography. The aneurysm will appear as a segment which does not move (akinetic) or bulges out paradoxically during systole (dyskinetic). Surgery is indicated if there is persistent heart failure, angina, uncontrollable ventricular arrhythmias or systemic emboli. Aneurysm resection may be combined with coronary bypass surgery.

Answer 1.16

(a) This man had cardiogenic shock secondary to a myocardial infarction. The diagnosis of cardiogenic shock is made by the reduced cardiac index (cardiac output corrected for surface area), the raised right heart filling pressure and the raised peripheral resistance (low cardiac output with underperfusion of tissues). Anaerobic metabolism occurs with increase in blood lactate.

(b) The physical signs are low blood pressure, raised pulse rate, possibly with an arrhythmia, cold and cyanosed periphery, raised jugular venous pressure, sweating, possible mental confusion and a urine output of less than 30 ml/h.

(c) The essentials of treatment include oxygen, analgesics and an intravenous diuretic such as frusemide. Anti-arrhythmic drugs may be indicated. Corticosteroids such as methylprednisolone or dextramethasone and an α-blocking drug are now frequently used, and if they induce a fall in the right heart filling pressure and total peripheral resistance are followed by intravenous fluid to keep the right atrial pressure in the normal range. If these measures fail an aortic balloon catheter may be indicated.

Answer 1.17

These findings are compatible with the diagnosis of rheumatic carditis. The elevated ASOT indicates a recent β-haemolytic streptococcal infection. The tachycardia and prolonged PR interval (normal not more than 0.2 seconds) substantiated a carditis.

These features are also compatible with a streptococcal infection in a patient with pre-existing heart block or on quinidine therapy.

Answer 1.18

(a) The differential diagnosis lies between a further myocardial infarction or the development of the postinfarction (Dressler's) syndrome.

(b) Further ECGs and cardiac enzyme measurements are needed. If the ECG is unchanged or shows changes of pericarditis then the prognosis is good although further attacks may occur. Cardiac enzymes will be elevated in either condition.

Answer 1.19

(*a*) The data are compatible with the diagnosis of a left atrial myxoma or subacute bacterial endocarditis (SBE). There are insufficient facts given to take the diagnosis further but blood cultures may establish SBE. Even if cultures are sterile the diagnosis is not excluded and a trial of antibiotics may be appropriate. An arterial embolus does not distinguish between the two as either myxomatous tissue or fragments of infected material may become detached.

(*b*) Echocardiography may well be helpful in demonstrating either a valvular defect or the presence of a filling defect in an atrium – most commonly the left.

Answer 1.20

(*a*) This patient had a third degree heart block; there is complete dissociation between the P waves (atrial rate) and the QRS complexes (ventricular rate).

(*b*) An artificial pacemaker should be inserted.

Answer 1.21

(*a*) There are retrograde P waves present and the rate is 45/ second. In addition there is ST depression. This was therefore a junctional bradycardia.

(*b*) This may be seen in digoxin toxicity and in this example sinus rhythm returned upon reducing the dose of digoxin.

Answer 1.22

(*a*) The ST segment is elevated in V2–V6 with deep Q waves in the same leads.

(*b*) This is the ECG of an acute extensive anterior transmural infarction.

(*c*) Predisposing factors include hyperlipidaemia, hypertension, use of the contraceptive pill, diabetes mellitus, cigarette smoking and a positive family history.

Answer 1.23

This rhythm strip shows a 2:1 heart block (sino-atrial block). The ventricular rate is 48 and the atrial rate 96 per minute.

Answer 1.24

There are no P waves, the QRS complexes are broadened and are merging with the T waves. All are features of hyperkalaemia. The plasma potassium was 8.3 mmol/l (mEq/1) in this man.

Answer 1.25

(*a*) This rhythm strip shows an atrial flutter with varying block – 1:1 to 1:3. The 'saw-tooth' flutter waves obscure the isoelectric line.
(*b*) Underlying causes include ischaemic heart disease, hyperthyroidism and rheumatic heart disease.
(*c*) The patient should be digitalized. This blocks A–V transmission of some of the atrial impulses, with slowing of the ventricular rate. In addition the flutter may return to sinus rhythm and the digoxin may then be withdrawn.

Answer 1.26

(*a*) This trace is an example of sinus bradycardia and sinus arrythmia.
(*b*) Sinus bradycardia is a normal finding in young people and athletes. It is also found in association with digoxin treatment, β-blockade therapy, hypothermia, obstructive jaundice, hypothyroidism and raised intracranial pressure.

Answer 1.27

(*a*) (*i*) There is an RSR' pattern in leads V4–V6, the S waves in leads V1–V3 are deep slurred and in V4–V6 notched with ST depression; and there is T wave inversion in leads V4–V6.
   (*ii*) The S wave in V1 plus the R wave in V5 is 40 mm.

(*b*) The features described in (*i*) are indicative of left bundle branch block. The trace is always pathological and may be found in ischaemic heart disease, hypertension, aortic valvular disease and following cardiac surgery. Left ventricular hypertrophy is indicated by (*ii*).

Answer 1.28

(*a*) This rhythm strip shows a second degree heart block (Wenckebach type).
(*b*) The ST elevation indicates a recent infarction but its site and extent cannot be stated from a rhythm strip alone.

Answer 1.29

(a) This rhythm strip shows atrial fibrillation with ventricular extra-systoles. There is an R on T phenomenon and the final portion of the strip shows ventricular fibrillation.

(b) Treatment includes: closed chest massage; intubation and 100% oxygen administration; setting up a drip; intravenous lignocaine; intravenous bicarbonate; DC shock.

Answer 1.30

(a) These chest leads show a complete right bundle branch block.

(b) There is an RSR′ pattern in leads V1–V3 and wide slurred S waves in leads V5 and V6.

(c) Right bundle branch may be found in: normal people; pulmonary embolism; chronic lung disease leading to right ventricular hypertrophy; congenital heart disease such as ASD; ischaemic heart disease; hypertensive heart disease; rheumatic heart disease; postcardiac surgery.

Answer 1.31

(a) and (b) The ST segment is elevated concave upwards in leads V2–V6. These are the classical findings of acute pericarditis. The ST elevation of an acute infarction is concave downwards.

(c) The patient is likely to have had central chest pain similar to that experienced with ischaemic heart disease. Pericardial pain tends to show postural variation while that of ischaemic heart disease does not.

Answer 1.32

(a) The strip shows ventricular bigeminy. Apart from the ventricular beats the other complexes are normal.

(b) This ECG finding may be found in: apparently normal people; ischaemic heart disease; digoxin toxicity; cardiomyopathies.

Answer 1.33

(a) This ECG strip shows a supraventricular tachycardia with bundle branch block. There is a rapid sequence of regular complexes (rate 165) and the QRS is widened which is not infrequent during rapid supra-ventricular rhythms resulting from either aberrant conduction or bundle branch block. The last 3 QRS complexes show a sinus tachycardia.

(*b*) Attacks may often be aborted by carotid sinus massage or by the Valsalva manoeuvre.

(*c*) Resistant cases may respond to digoxin or practolol alone or combined. Verapamil may be used but if so should not be used with β-blockers. Cardioversion may be required.

Answer 1.34

There is an S wave in leads V1–V6 indicating clockwise rotation. The ST segment is depressed in leads V4–V6 and the T wave is asymmetrically inverted in the same leads. This is an ischaemic trace but without evidence of infarction.

Answer 1.35

The first two complexes are normal; there are then four different beats. The four abnormal beats are regular and are supraventricular in origin. The P wave is buried in the T wave of the preceding complex and the QRS is different, implying aberrant conduction. As there are more than three consecutive extrasystoles, by definition this constitutes a tachycardia. The diagnosis is therefore supraventricular tachycardia with aberrant conduction.

Answer 1.36

(*a*) This rhythm is atrial fibrillation as shown by the absence of P waves and the total irregularity of the QRS complexes.

(*b*) The most common causes are ischaemic heart disease and hyperthyroidism. Other causes include rheumatic heart disease, cardiomyopathy, constrictive pericarditis, acute fevers, post-thoracotomy, infiltration of the pericardium with tumours and pulmonary embolism. In addition a congenital form and an idiopathic or lone form are described. If there is a predisposing cause atrial fibrillation is more likely to occur with advancing age.

Answer 1.37

(*a*) This trace shows a wandering pacemaker. The ventricular rate is constant but the P waves vary, becoming biphasic and inverted with shortening of the PR interval. The term 'wandering pacemaker' is considered by some to be a misnomer as the rhythm is dual, both sino-atrial (SA) and arteriovenous (AV) nodes discharging spontaneously with variable asynchronism.

(b) This condition may be found by chance in healthy individuals but is also associated with digoxin therapy. In the latter circumstance the dose should be reduced.

Answer 1.38

This man had heart failure. The normal arm—tongue time is 10–16 seconds when saccharine is given as a rapid intravenous bolus. In circulatory conditions where the rate of venous blood flow is reduced, the time for an intravenous injection of a tasteable substance to reach the tongue is increased.

Answer 1.39

There is a tachycardia and the T waves are symmetrically peaked. This may be a normal trace taken from a person with a thin chest wall or it may be associated with early hyperkalaemia. One should not rely upon an ECG to diagnose hyperkalaemia as hyperkalaemic changes may only become apparent at a dangerously high plasma potassium concentration or may never develop.

Answer 1.40

This is an example of a paced ECG. The pacing 'spikes' immediately precede the QRS complex, which is widened. This example was taken from a patient with a permanent pacemaker, the 'spike' from a temporary pacemaker being smaller.

Answer 1.41

(a) There is a tachycardia, the rate being about 200/minute. Each QRS complex is approximately equal in dimensions and the width represents more than 0.12 seconds (3 small squares at the standard 25 mm speed of ECG paper). The QRS complexes are abnormal and dissociated P waves are present. These are all features of a ventricular tachycardia.

(b) A diagnostic feature (not shown) would be the presence of 'capture beats' — normal beats found amongst the tachycardia beats.

Answer 2.1

(*a*) The clue to this diagnosis comes from the agglutination of the red blood cells; this suggests that cold agglutins were present. This finding occurs in more than 50% of patients with *Mycoplasma pneumoniae* infection.
(*b*) The diagnosis is substantiated by demonstrating:

(*i*) a positive complement fixation test to *M. pneumoniae;*
(*ii*) the presence of cold haemagglutins.

The absence of a leucocytosis and pathogenic bacteria in the sputum helps initially to distinguish this condition from a bacterial pneumonia.
(*c*) The treatment is tetracycline 2 g daily for 10 days.

Answer 2.2

(*a*) There was hypoxaemia, hypercapnia and acidosis. In Britain these are typical findings when arterial blood is sampled from a patient with an acute exacerbation of chronic bronchitis.
(*b*) With resolution of the acute state the oxygen tension rises to about 70–90 mmHg (9.0–12.0 kPa) and the carbon dioxide falls to about 50 mmHg (6.6 kPa). There is a considerable variation from patient to patient. Between exacerbations of acute and chronic bronchitis the blood pH is usually within the normal range.

Answer 2.3

(*a*) and (*b*) The sweat sodium was equivocal and would have to be repeated. A level of less than 40 mmol/l is normal and more than 70 mmol/l is abnormal. The serum IgA was low (normal range 0.4–1.45 g/l for a child of this age); secretory IgA may well be low also. Frequent respiratory infections are a recognized problem in such patients. There is no specific therapy; each respiratory episode is treated as required.

Answer 2.4

(*a*) This man had an obstructive pattern of lung disease such as is found in chronic bronchitis.

(b) The FEV_1 (1.3 litres) and the FVC (2.5 litres) are much reduced. The FEV_1/FVC ratio is 52%. In normal people the ratio is 70–80%. FEV_1 is reduced because of high airways resistance. The low FVC is due to airways closing with limitation of expiration.

(c) If this trace were obtained when the patient had no exacerbation of chronic bronchitis the arterial pH would probably have been normal, but hypoxaemia and hypercapnoea tend to persist.

Answer 2.5

(a) This spirogram is typical of restrictive lung disease.

(b) The FEV_1/FVC ratio is $3/3.5 \times 100 = 86\%$. In health the FEV_1 should be at least 70–80% of the FVC.

(c) In a normal man aged 39 years the FEV_1 should be about 4.5 litres and the FVC 5.7 litres, giving a ratio of 79%. In this patient the ratio is supranormal. This is because the FVC is reduced but the FEV_1 is not proportionately reduced. The ratio therefore rises.

Answer 2.6

(a) This is a restrictive pattern of lung disease $(2.8/3.1 \times 100 = 90\%)$. Such a pattern is found in ankylosing spondylosis. There is no increased airways resistance but movements of the thoracic cage are restricted so the FVC is reduced and the ratio FEV_1/FVC is supranormal.

(b) About 90% of such patients possess HLA B27.

Answer 2.7

(a) There was a combined respiratory and metabolic acidosis with hypoxaemia.

(b) The infant was premature both in terms of gestational age and of birth weight, and the likely diagnosis was therefore respiratory distress syndrome. The respiratory rate might well have been rising before the occurrence of the cyanotic attack. The incidence of major congenital abnormalities is higher in low birth weight babies and has to be considered. Such abnormalities include congenital heart disease, tracheo-oesophageal fistula and diaphragmatic hernia. Also inhalation of regurgitated stomach contents may give rise to a similar clinical and biochemical picture.

(c) A chest X-ray is essential. Respiratory distress syndrome will be confirmed by the typical ground glass appearance with an air bronchogram. Diaphragmatic hernia will be obvious if present. In a case of congenital heart disease abnormalities of size, shape and position of the heart and of the degree of vascularity of the lungs may be diagnostically useful. Patchy consolidation due to inhalation will also be demonstrated.

Answer 2.8

(*a*) This patient had hypoxaemia with a low normal P_{CO_2}. Two conditions which produce these findings are moderate pulmonary thrombo-embolism and lobar pneumonia.

(*b*) A large area of lung is not available for oxygen transfer, hence the hypoxaemia. As the reserve capacity for CO_2 transport is greater, the P_{CO_2} is normal or reduced if there is tachypnoea. The failure of the P_{O_2} to increase following approximate doubling of the inspired oxygen concentration is due to imbalance between perfusion and ventilation of the diseased area. The area is perfused but not oxygenated in lobar pneumonia and neither perfused nor oxygenated following pulmonary infarction. The functional effect is the same.

Answer 2.9

This man had late-onset intrinsic asthma as shown by the reduced peak flow rate, the obstructive FEV_1/FVC ratio which partially responds to isoprenaline and the sputum eosinophils. A circulating eosinophilia may also be present.

Answer 2.10

(*a*) Aneurysm of the descending aorta, paravertebral abscess and neurogenic tumours such as neurofibromas, neurolemmomas and neuroblastomas occur in area A.

(*b*) A retrosternal thyroid is found in area B and occasionally an aneurysm of the innominate artery. An hiatus hernia is the major cause of a mass in area C; achalasia of a cardia with dilatation of the oesophagus could produce a similar appearance. A pericardial cyst is seen in area D.

Answer 2.11

(*a*) This patient had a diffusion defect. Before exercise while the partial pressure of oxygen was normal, partial pressure of carbon dioxide was subnormal. The lower limit of P_{CO_2} is 36 mmHg (4.8 kPa). This example is characteristic of a moderate loss of diffusion capacity. These patients have to hyperventilate to maintain a normal partial pressure of oxygen and in so doing 'wash out' carbon dioxide and the partial pressure of carbon dioxide becomes subnormal.

(b) Following exercise, the demand for oxygen exceeds the ability of the lung to deliver oxygen and the partial pressure falls. With tachypnoea the wash-out effect upon carbon dioxide increases, the $P\text{co}_2$ falls further and the patient becomes alkalotic (arterial pH 7.53 in this example).

(c) The transfer factor T_{CO} (D_{CO}) should be measured to confirm the diagnosis. It would be reduced by at least 50% of the predicted value in this case and would not rise with exercise.

Answer 2.12

(a) This curve was obtained from a healthy person.

(b) This patient had severe air trapping with consequent persistent hyperinflated lungs. The tidal volume (inner curve) is considerably larger than the normal and the maximum respiratory exertion (outer curve) is much distorted. These measurements were obtained from a patient with advanced interstitial pulmonary fibrosis.

Answer 2.13

(i) The low blood oxygen and the normal CO_2 concentration make this a Type I pattern of respiratory failure. This is most frequently seen in an acute asthmatic attack.

(ii) These blood gas concentrations are also compatible with 'shock', e.g. systemic hypotension before hypercapnia has developed.

Answer 2.14

This patient should have the following measurements:

(i) Sweat sodium.
(ii) The plasma level of α_1-antitrypsin.

Using the pilocarpine iontophoresis method of stimulating local sweating in patients with cystic fibrosis the concentration of sodium and chloride in the sweat is more than 70 mmol/l (mEq/1). The normal sweat sodium is less than 40 mmol/l.

α_1-antitrypsin deficiency is associated with the early development of emphysema in a few patients which may then become complicated with recurrent chest infections and further lung damage. The explanation for this enzyme deficiency and the development of emphysema is unknown. The diagnosis of the deficiency may be of value in genetic counselling.

Answer 2.15

(*a*) Precipitating factors must be sought from the history — exposure to mouldy hay would be particularly relevant in this man.
(*b*) The diagnosis was an acute Farmer's lung or extrinsic allergic alveolitis.
(*c*) The condition develops in some people 4—8 hours after inhalation of spores of *Micropolyspora faeni*.
(*d*) This patient had a restrictive pattern of lung function with hypoxaemia and reduced gas transfer.
(*e*) The disease is mediated by a Type III (Gell and Coombes') or Arthus immunological mechanism which is dependent upon complement, circulating antibody (not IgE) and inhaled antigen. Local complexes form.
(*f*) Treatment of the acute phase is with prednisolone. Long-term treatment is by the avoidance of mouldy hay and hence spores or if not feasible the use of a respirator while handling the hay.

Answer 2.16

(*a*) The blood gas tensions fit an acute exacerbation of chronic bronchitis but the pH is very low and bicarbonate is too low for a respiratory acidosis. The figures are those of both respiratory and non-respiratory acidosis.
(*b*) The patient required urgent investigation for causes of non-respiratory acidosis — diabetic ketoacidosis, lactic acidosis (*see* Answer 6.12, page 144), aspirin poisoning and failure to secrete hydrogen ion due to acute or acute on chronic respiratory failure. This man had taken an overdose of aspirin tablets as his chest condition was deteriorating.

Answer 2.17

(*a*) This man should be considered to have *Pneumocystis carinii* infection and treated as such without delay.
(*b*) The patient should be bronchoscoped and scrapings taken which might demonstrate the parasite. Sputum should also be examined for tubercule bacilli.
(*c*) Regardless of the bronchoscopic findings the patient should receive intramuscular pentamidine and oral septrin. Withdrawal of prednisolone and azathioprine may be necessary. *P. carinii* infection has a high mortality and it is better to lose the transplant kidney and save the patient than to lose both.

Answer 2.18

(*a*) This patient had Caplan's syndrome. The diagnosis is made from the following features:

(*i*) The radiological appearance described in the question.

(*ii*) The patient is a miner (the condition appears to be most frequent in South Wales).

(*iii*) The presence of rheumatoid arthritis (the positive Rose—Waaler test).

(*iv*) Minimal or no evidence of pneumoconiosis.

Caplan's syndrome is multiple rheumatoid nodules in the lungs of miners who have or who will develop joint manifestations of rheumatoid arthritis. Conversely the joint lesions may precede the lung disease by years.

(*b*) While the FEV_1 and FVC are often reduced in these patients, it is a reflection upon co-existing chronic bronchitis and detailed lung function in these patients shows no specific physiological defect as would be expected.

(*c*) There is no relation between Caplan's syndrome and progressive massive fibrosis (PMF). PMF is classified as a complicated pneumoconiosis in which there are only one or two opacities per lung which gradually enlarge, becoming round or oval, and may occupy almost a whole lobe. In the remaining lung fields there are substantial simple pneumoconiotic changes. These patients do not have rheumatoid arthritis. The two conditions are quite separate but both occur in miners.

Answer 2.19

(*a*) The figures were those of an acute respiratory alkalosis although the Po_2 was low. This was expected as a tachypnoea was present.

(*b*) The differential diagnosis includes the following:

(*i*) Multiple pulmonary emboli – not infrequent following pelvic surgery in fat women.

(*ii*) Haemorrhage – the Hb was 8.7 g/dl.

(*iii*) Disseminated intravascular coagulation – causing the 'shock lung' (adult respiratory distress syndrome).

The data given in this question do not allow further analysis of this woman's condition.

Answer 3.1

This ascitic albumin concentration is in the transudate range and is found in cirrhosis, nephrotic syndrome and congestive cardiac failure. However in some cases of congestive cardiac failure the ascitic albumin concentration may be up to 50 g/l (5.0 g/100 ml).

Other causes of ascitic fluid — malignancy, tuberculous or bacterial peritonitis — or fluid found in association with acute pancreatitis have albumin concentrations in the exudative range (more than 25 g/l (2.5 mg/100 ml)).

Answer 3.2

(*a*) It is very probable that this woman had primary biliary cirrhosis because itching is a common presenting feature of these patients (who are characteristically middle aged) and mitochondrial antibodies are found in 90% of cases. These antibodies are directed against the inner lining of the cristae of mitochondria.

(*b*) A liver biopsy will show mononuclear cell infiltration with accumulation into lymphoid follicles and bile duct injury and destruction.

Answer 3.3

(*a*) These are the biochemical features of an active chronic hepatitis unassociated with antinuclear antibodies or the hepatitis B antigen. The piecemeal necrosis of the liver helps to differentiate the condition from primary biliary cirrhosis.

(*b*) The condition will respond, at least initially, to corticosteroids but there is a distinct probability of subsequent development of cirrhosis and perhaps portal hypertension and liver failure.

Answer 3.4

(*a*) The diagnosis from these data is that of an active hepatitic process.

(*b*) The second group of data fits only one diagnosis — that of active chronic (lupoid) hepatitis. The presence of a high titre of antinuclear and antismooth muscle antibodies with a high serum gamma globulin (which is chiefly IgG) and the absence of hepatitis B antigen make the diagnosis. High titres of rubella and measles antibodies are found in some of these patients also.

(c) The prognosis is very variable. The course is fluctuant and marked by episodes of deterioration when jaundice and malaise are prominent. This hepatitis is almost always progressive to a cirrhosis. Mortality is greatest in the first 2 years when the condition is most active. Steroids prolong life in the short term but most patients eventually die of hepatocellular failure with or without portal hypertension.

Answer 3.5

(a) This pattern of enzyme and bilirubin increase is often seen in association with hypersensitivity reactions involving the liver — an intrahepatic cholestatic jaundice. The normal serum albumin indicates that this is an acute type of lesion. In some patients a blood and hepatic eosinophilia may be found.

(b) The hepatic histology would show intact overall architecture with centrizonal bile stasis. Liver cells show patchy necrosis. The portal zones usually contain mononuclear cells and eosinophils. The bile ducts are of normal calibre.

(c) The most common cause of a sensitivity type cholestasis is chlorpromazine but it occurs in less than 0.5% of patients treated with this drug. Other phenothiazines may induce a similar hepatotoxicity. There are many other potential drugs in this category. They include: chlorpropamide, sulphonamides, erythromycin estolate, nitrofurantoin diphenylhydantoin and imipramine.

Answer 3.6

(a) The ^{14}C glycocholic acid breath test is a measure of bacterial overgrowth of intestinal bacteria. It is most frequently positive in patients who have had previous ileal resection or blind loop syndromes and is sometimes so in patients with liver disease. Bacterial deconjugation of the ^{14}C glycine from the cholic acid occurs excessively if (i) there is a bacterial overgrowth in a stagnant loop of gut; or (ii) there are normal gut bacteria but the enterohepatic circulation of conjugated bile salts is interrupted by ileal resection. In either of these circumstances release of ^{14}C from the cholic acid occurs and is measured as exhaled $^{14}CO_2$. The concentration of $^{14}CO_2$ is proportional to the amount of bacterial deconjugation of bile salts which has occurred.

(b) In this patient either a Pólya gastrectomy or an ileal resection had been conducted previously.

Answer 3.7

(*a*) This man was a chronic alcoholic. Such people have matutinal nausea and vomiting and bouts of diarrhoea. The hypochloraemia, hypokalaemia and alkalosis are thus explained. (*See* Answer 6.26, page 148 for a discussion of electrolyte changes following vomiting).

(*b*) The low blood urea is a reflection of the subnutritional state of alcoholics — wine and spirits contain only trivial quantities of protein and alcoholics need to spend available money on ethanol, not food.

Answer 3.8

(*a*) This patient had mild elevation of SGPT, SGOT, alkaline phosphatase and bilirubin. The SGOT elevation reflected the myocardial infarction but the alkaline phosphatase, bilirubin and to a lesser extent the SGPT represented liver damage. The most likely explanation of these abnormalities is venous congestion of the liver secondary to right heart failure.

(*b*) Treatment is the administration of a potent 'loop' diuretic and if atrial fibrillation is present digoxin is indicated. With the control of the heart failure in this patient liver discomfort disappeared and the liver function tests became normal in 3 days.

Answer 3.9

(*a*) This man had disseminated intravascular coagulation (consumption coagulopathy). There was a low (and perhaps falling) platelet count. Plasma fibrinogen was low (normal 0.2–0.4 g/l) which was reflected by the raised titre of fibrinogen degeneration products (consumed fibrinogen). As this man had recent urgent bowel surgery it must be presumed that he had a Gram-negative septicaemia and that the disseminated intravascular coagulation was secondary to the infection.

(*b*) The major complications are usually seen together: bleeding, hypotension from the 'shock' of septicaemia and varying degrees of renal impairment. Jaundice is not infrequent and worsens the prognosis.

Answer 3.10

The problem was one of hypo-albuminaemia with normal hepatic function and no proteinuria. This suggests either malabsorption or loss of protein from the gut lesion. Progressive anorexia is a common feature of carcinoma of the stomach and occasionally some of these tumours exude protein to an extent sufficient to cause hypo-albuminaemia.

The laboratory figures in this example together with the anorexia favour a gastric tumour more than malabsorption as malabsorption symptoms are usually those of diarrhoea, abdominal discomfort and flatulence.

Answer 3.11

(*a*) This man had steatorrhoea, as shown by the increased faecal fat excretion. The most likely diagnosis was the reintroduction of gluten either by relaxing the diet or by accidentally taking gluten. The other possibility was the development of small bowel lymphomata.

(*b*) The diagnosis of gluten reintroduction is made by history. A detailed dietary history taken by a dietition may be needed. A small bowel lymphoma is diagnosed by small bowel radiography and subsequent open biopsy.

Answer 3.12

The important point in this case is to appreciate that the ascites was not due to hepatocellular dysfunction. Ascites of liver origin is always associated with hypo-albuminaemia. The peak flow rate suggests no serious lung disease; the low blood pressure and soft heart sounds suggest constrictive pericarditis which is a well recognized cause of ascites.

Answer 3.13

(*a*) This woman had acute pancreatitis as shown by the hyperglycaemia, the hypocalcaemia and the presence of methaemalbuminaemia. The methaemalbuminaemia results from tryptic digestion of extravasated blood around the pancreas.

(*b*) Important additional investigations are the measurement of serum and urinary amylase and arterial pH. Increase in amylase may be transient and is not specific for pancreatitis as it is elevated in perforated ulcer and intestinal obstruction although the increases rarely approach the levels found in pancreatitis.

(*c*) An erect abdominal X-ray should be taken to aid exclusion of a perforated ulcer. If the woman survives, gallstones should be excluded. In Britain gallstones are found in 50–60% of cases of acute pancreatitis.

Answer 3.14

This man was an example of the Zollinger–Ellison syndrome (non-beta cell tumour of the pancreas). A basal secretion of 17 mmol/h of hydrogen ions is very high (normal basal H^+ secretion 0.5–5.0 mmol/h) and no increase follows pentagastrin injection as the patient's condition is due to excess endogenous gastrin production. Plasma gastrin can be assayed by a radioimmunoassay and fasting concentrations may be 25 times above normal. The Zollinger–Ellison syndrome may be associated with functioning adenomas of other endocrine organs – parathyroids, pituitary and adrenal – the polyglandular syndrome. The most common association of the Zollinger–Ellison syndrome is with the parathyroid glands.

Answer 3.15

None of the data provide a contraindication to portovenous anastomosis except for the positive morphia provocation test. This implies that the hepatic ability to metabolize morphia is significantly impaired and portosystemic encephalopathy might follow the operation. However portosystemic encephalopathy may well be considered better than death due to variceal bleeding.

Answer 3.16

There was macrocytosis, hypocalcaemia and mild hypo-albuminaemia. In all three questions the differential diagnosis lies between malabsorption from the gut or dietary insufficiency.

(a) In the Caucasian child coeliac disease is the most likely cause giving rise to these findings.
(b) Some immigrant children receive inadequate diets and as in children with malabsorption they have iron deficiency anaemias in addition.
(c) In a woman aged 41 years, one would expect a malabsorption from the data given.

Answer 3.17

These findings could occur in:

(a) coeliac disease, post-gastroenteritis and disaccharidase deficiency.
(b) coeliac disease, dermatitis herpetiformis, Zollinger–Ellison syndrome and in some cases of tropical sprue.

Answer 3.18

(*a*) The child was very small for her age (assuming that the birth weight was average). There was evidence of malabsorption from the xylose test. Macrocytic anaemia may also be a feature of malabsorption. Stool tryptic activity is a rather unreliable and non-specific test for malabsorption.

(*b*) A sweat test and jejunal biopsy are necessary to diagnose cystic fibrosis and coeliac disease respectively. The presence of reducing substances in the stools would be evidence of sugar malabsorption and specific sugar tolerance tests could be undertaken to elucidate that aspect.

Answer 3.19

(*a*) The baby had unconjugated hyperbilirubinaemia without significant anaemia and normal liver cell function. It would be necessary to check the mother's blood group – if O Rhesus positive, ABO incompatibility would be likely. The Coombs' test is usually negative and detection of abnormal anti-A in the mother is not always possible.

(*b*) If there is no blood group incompatibility, breast milk jaundice should be considered. Evidence of infection should be sought especially if the baby appears unwell; among the investigations the urine must be cultured. If the jaundice were to persist hypothyroidism or galactosaemia should be considered.

(*c*) Treatment includes: adequate fluid intake, temporary withdrawal of breast milk and phototherapy until a sustained fall in bilirubin is achieved.

Answer 3.20

(*a*) The hyperbilirubinaemia is conjugated and the results suggest cholestasis. This might be due to conditions giving rise to 'neonatal hepatitis' or to biliary atresia. The abnormalities of liver function found in the two groups overlap considerably. The α-fetoprotein is significantly raised (normal 10–40 μg/ml in children). This is in favour of hepatitis: it is low in biliary obstruction. In biliary atresia 5-nucleotidase concentrations are raised.

(*b*) (*i*) ^{131}I Rose Bengal excretion test – stool excretion is less than 10% in biliary atresia.

(*ii*) Percutaneous liver biopsy – this should only be performed if the coagulation profile is normal. The histology may not always be diagnostic.

(*iii*) Operative cholangiography is indicated where other results suggest atresia.

(*iv*) When the results are equivocal a trial of therapy with cholestyramine to promote bile secretion and flow may be used. Failure to improve would indicate atresia.

Answer 3.21

There was a high bilirubin in the presence of a normal alkaline phosphatase and modestly elevated liver enzymes. The alkaline phosphatase concentration virtually excluded an obstructive lesion. The most likely diagnosis was postoperative jaundice associated with infection. Halothane hepatitis is also possible but assuming this patient had been anaesthetized with this drug for the first time icterus on the fourth postoperative day would be early. Also with a hepatitis, liver enzymes tend to be more elevated and the prothrombin time more prolonged.

The differential diagnosis includes a previously unrecognized cirrhosis and an interhepatic abscess.

Answer 3.22

(*a*) This man had polycythaemia rubra vera. The sudden abdominal symptoms with mild jaundice and raised liver enzymes are suggestive of a development of hepatic venous obstruction (Budd–Chiari syndrome). One would expect enlargement of the liver and ascites to develop.

(*b*) The Budd–Chiari syndrome is an occasional complication of polycythaemia rubra vera but in many cases the aetiology is unexplained.

(*c*) The generally poor uptake of isotope by the liver is to be expected; in some people the caudate lobe may have venous drainage to the infradiaphragmatic portion of the inferior vena cava other than by one of the main hepatic veins. It may therefore be spared during a thrombotic episode and excess isotope will accumulate in this region.

(*d*) An inferior vena cavagram is indicated to demonstrate a characteristic narrowing distortion of the vein throughout its intrahepatic course.

Answer 3.23

(*a*) This woman had hypercupriuria, hypercupraemia and a raised liver copper concentration. The raised copper concentrations are suggestive of Wilson's disease but the normal concentration of ceruloplasmin is much against this diagnosis. The mild jaundice and mild elevation of alanine transaminase with a very raised alkaline phosphatase in a middle-aged woman is very suggestive of primary biliary cirrhosis.

(*b*) This would be confirmed by finding a high titre of antimicrosomal antibodies. This antibody is present in a serum of about 95% of patients with primary biliary cirrhosis.

Answer 3.24

(*a*) This patient had a mild hyperbilirubinaemia in the absence of any abnormality of hepatic cellular function, haemolytic jaundice or obstruction to bile drainage. One has to consider the familial or constitutional hyperbilirubinaemias. In this case there was no evidence for the Dublin–Johnson type in which the hyperbilirubinaemia may be much greater and the BSP retention test is abnormal. Liver biopsy of this condition shows normal architecture with an excess of an abnormal pigment which resembles melanin. The Rotor type of hyperbilirubinaemia is biochemically very similar to the Dublin–Johnson but the liver biopsy is not pigmented. The Crigler–Najjar hyperbilirubinaemia presents in childhood and a diagnosis would not have been delayed to the age of 40 years as in this case. The very rare primary shunt hyperbilirubinaemia is associated with very high levels of urinary urobilinogen and reticulocytosis may be present.

The data presented here are compatible with Gilbert's hyperbilirubinaemia in which the only abnormality is a mild elevation of total bilirubin.

(*b*) A liver biopsy is not indicated.

(*c*) If patients with Gilbert's disease are fasted for 36–48 hours plasma bilirubin tends to rise further which gives some confirmation of the diagnosis in this condition which is entirely benign.

Answer 3.25

(*a*) This woman had hypophosphataemia, hyperglycaemia and hypokalaemic alkalosis. The symptoms and biochemical findings are found in patients who are being fed intravenously with concentrated dextrose solutions especially those who are already nutritionally depleted.

(*b*) The symptoms are due to the hypophosphataemia which is more marked if additional insulin is given. Hypophosphataemia is very probably due to the rapid acceleration of glucose phosphorylation induced by dextrose infusion with consequent cellular uptake of inorganic phosphorus from the plasma. The hypokalaemic alkalosis is a reflection upon rapid cellular uptake of circulating potassium.

(*c*) In parenteral nutrition concentrated sugar solutions are essential for energy requirements. Phosphate, additional to that available in intravenous lipid preparations, should be given so that the patient receives about 0.5–0.7 mmol (mEq) phosphate/kg bodyweight daily.

Answer 3.26

All the data were abnormal and the most simple explanation is malabsorption of protein, calcium and iron leading to a low urea, calcium, albumin and an anaemia and with the development of osteomalacia.

Similar figures would also be obtained with severe liver disease with associated gut bleeding.

Answer 3.27

Raised IgM and positive antimitochondrial antibodies are very constant features of primary biliary cirrhosis. They are also found in chronic active hepatitis but this condition is rarely associated with a neutral or alkaline pH (renal tubular acidosis) when there is a 60% association between primary biliary cirrhosis and renal tubular acidosis. Haematemesis secondary to oesophageal varices occurs in almost half the patients with primary biliary cirrhosis and occurs relatively early in the disease – during the first 2 years from onset.

Answer 4.1

This man was oliguric: $15 \times 24 = 360$ ml of urine per day. The oliguria was consequent upon dehydration. The high urine osmolarity, the U/P osm ratio of 2.37 ($700 \div 295$) and the low urinary sodium indicate normal renal response to fluid deprivation. The raised urea is a reflection upon the dehydration and in the presence of oliguria urea clearance falls. The serum osmolarity is at the upper limit of normal. Given adequate hydration the blood urea will return to normal.

Answer 4.2

(a) The creatinine clearance is calculated from the formula $\dfrac{UV}{P}$ where U = urine excretion of creatinine, V = volume of urine per minute, P = plasma concentration of creatinine.

Hence, using molar concentrations: $\dfrac{25}{140} \times \dfrac{1200}{1400} = 149$ ml/min;

and using mass concentrations: $\dfrac{2825}{1.6} \times \dfrac{1200}{1440} = 147$ ml/min.

Normal creatinine clearance is about 120 ml/min (the GFR is 127 ml per min per 1.7 m²).
(b) In the above example the creatinine clearance is above normal. There is also a 'heavy' proteinuria of 22 g/day. Occasionally creatinine clearance is supranormal in the presence of a heavy proteinuria. This is because 'excess' of creatinine is lost into the urine. There are two mechanisms by which this arises:

(i) Increased tubular secretion of creatinine.
(ii) Reduced oncotic pressure at glomerular level due to a reduced serum albumin which allows increased quantities of creatinine to pass the glomerulus. Hypo-albuminaemia accompanies a proteinuria of 22 g/day.

Answer 4.3

The daily weight gain, reduced plasma volume, the hypercholesterolaemia, hyperaldosteronism (upper limit of normal 330 pmol/l), serum albumin of 27 g/l and a daily proteinuria of 12–19 g are all usual features of nephrotic syndrome and have no prognostic significance.
Adverse features are the presence of purpura and hypertension.

Favourable features are: nephrotic syndrome at the age of 5 — the majority of such children will have the minimal change glomerular lesion which usually has a very good prognosis — and highly selective proteinuria of 0.01 in a child. In an adult proteinuria may be selective but is not necessarily related to a good prognosis.

The hypocalcuria is a usual feature of the early stages of nephrotic syndrome and is of no significance prognostically. If still present after say 6 weeks hypocalcuria would imply persistence of sodium and water retention and hence severe nephrotic syndrome.

The reduced C3 (normal range 0.1–0.18 g/l (120–180 mg/100 ml)) is very probably an adverse feature and while not adequately interpretable on its own, would suggest a membranoproliferative glomerulonephritis (mesangiocapillary glomerulonephritis). However hypocomplementaemia occurs in acute glomerulonephritis which may present with nephrotic syndrome and may have an excellent prognosis in a child.

Answer 4.4

There was a renal artery stenosis of the kidney which was drained by catheter B. The urine volume and sodium excretion are decreased from that kidney while the excretion of urea and para-amino hippurate (PAH) is increased. These are the biochemical features of a functionally important renal artery stenosis. Because of the decreased blood flow in the kidney which is supplied by the stenosed artery there is 'more' time available for sodium reabsorption and also for excretion of urea, creatinine and exogenous substances such as PAH.

Answer 4.5

There was a large quantity of protein and glucose in the urine. The normal urine protein excretion is not more than 200 mg/day and normal glucose excretion measured by the oxidase method is 50–300 mg daily. This man was a diabetic and had developed nephrotic syndrome which was shown to be due to the development of the Kimmelstiel–Wilson lesion.

Answer 4.6

(a) Marked fluid retention, hypo-albuminaemia and a highly selective renal clearance for plasma proteins strongly suggest that this child had

122

a minimal change glomerulonephritis ('no light change' glomerulonephritis). Children have a tendency to retain fluid within the abdomen as well as peripherally and ascites is not normally a feature of an adult with nephrotic syndrome.

(b) The treatment of choice is prednisolone with which a rapid cessation of the proteinuria usually occurs. Occasionally cyclophosphamide has to be used but because of potential gonadal damage should be reserved for patients in whom steroids cannot be used or in whom steroid side-effects limit dosage.

(c) The characteristic course of minimal change glomerulonephritis is one of relapse and remission. Treatment almost certainly induces remission of the condition more rapidly than no treatment but the process may remit without any drugs. Highly selective proteinuria indicates a highly probable steroid-induced remission.

Answer 4.7

(a) This patient had osteomalacia.

(b) The normal concentration of 25-OHD$_3$ indicates adequate dietary vitamin D and normal hepatic hydroxylation of vitamin D$_3$. The very low 1,25-di-OHD$_3$ and 24,25-di-OHD$_3$ indicate failure of adequate hydroxylation of 25-OHD$_3$. This patient had therefore severe renal disease because 25-OHD$_3$ is hydroxylated in the kidney. Chronicity of the renal disease is implied by the development of 'renal osteomalacia' (renal osteodystrophy). The grossly raised parathormone level was a reflection upon chronic hypocalcaemia which is a very constant feature of chronic renal failure.

(c) The serum phosphate will lie in the range of 2.0–4.0 mmol/l (6–13 mg/100 ml) or more. Serum urate is likely to be 0.5–0.7 mmol/l (8–12 mg/100 ml) or more. These figures are simply a reflection upon chronic renal failure and are not related to the disorded 25-OHD$_3$ metabolism.

Answer 4.8

(a) Haematuria of glomerular origin in an adolescent is likely to be an expression of one of four nephritides: Berger's C3/IgA (recurrent haematuria), Henoch–Schönlein purpura, membranoproliferative glomerulonephritis (mesangiocapillary glomerulonephritis) or acute post-streptococcal nephritis. In this question the discriminating features are a normal GFR, the very low protein excretion and the raised IgA. Berger's lesion is the only one of the four possibilities which usually has a normal GFR at presentation. It is also associated with minimal urinary protein loss and often with a raised serum IgA.

(b) The history should be expanded to include recent infections. Berger's nephritis often occurs at the height of or shortly after an upper respiratory tract infection and acute post-streptococcal nephritis has a latent interval of about 10–14 days following a streptococcal infection of the throat or skin. Acute post-streptococcal nephritis is now uncommon in Western Europe. Henoch–Schönlein nephritis tends to follow joint, skin and gut lesions.

Answer 4.9

(a) The three essential features of nephrotic syndrome are present: pitting oedema, 'heavy' proteinuria and hypo-albuminaemia. Note that raised plasma lipids are not essential for the diagnosis. Hyperlipidaemia has no constant relationship to hypo-albuminaemia in nephrotic syndrome. The urine sodium is much reduced – 16 mmol/24 h – while the plasma sodium is normal. This is a feature of an acute nephrotic – avid sodium retention as a result of secondary hyperaldosteronism. Sodium is stored extravascularly together with water and constitutes the pitting oedema. It should be emphasized that the nephrotic syndrome is not a diagnosis *per se* but a biochemical state. The underlying diagnosis is made by determining the renal morphology.

(b) The urinary aldosterone will be raised. The diminished circulating volume of nephrotic syndrome stimulates the renin–angiotensin axis and is one of the major factors causing diminished sodium excretion.

Answer 4.10

These figures are compatible with adult renal tubular acidosis (RTA) and can also be secondary to ureterosigmoidostomy. In RTA there is a failure to maintain the normal gradient of hydrogen ions across the distal renal tubules – hence the acidosis (reduced bicarbonate). The 'anion gap' left by the reduced bicarbonate is 'filled' by chloride ion. Normally sodium is exchanged for potassium or hydrogen ions in the distal renal tubules. In RTA there is insufficient hydrogen ion available and potassium is exchanged for sodium – hypokalaemia results. In ureterosigmoidostomy, chloride and hydrogen ions are well absorbed from the bowel with resulting hyperchloraemia and acidosis. Potassium is the major large bowel cation and is not reabsorbed to any extent. It is not known whether the hyperchloraemia reflects an excess loss by the kidney as a consequence of infection or whether the bowel secretes an excess of potassium due to a mucosal irritation by urine.

Answer 4.11

(*a*) These data indicate disease of the left kidney, but are not sufficient to specify its nature. The renal lesion is left sided because the renin excretion of the left kidney is higher than that from the right. To illustrate the cause of a unilateral renal disease an IVP (IVU) and perhaps aortography are indicated. Ureteric obstruction should also be excluded.

(*b*) The ratio of renin production is 2.2 (4.7 ÷ 2.1) L:R. It is generally held that hypertension may be cured or ameliorated if the ratio of renin production from a diseased and non-diseased kidney exceeds 1.5. From these data it appears that surgery would be beneficial.

Answer 4.12

(*a*) There is a discrepancy between the plasma creatinine which is approximately equivalent to a GFR of 10–15 ml/min and urea which very approximately is equivalent to a GFR of about 30–40 ml/min.

(*b*) This reduction in the urea/creatinine ratio is found in a patient in chronic renal failure after the introduction of a low protein diet. The GFR is unchanged but the protein and hence urea load to be excreted is reduced. Similar urea and creatinine figures are found after a period of haemodialysis or peritoneal dialysis. Either procedure removes urea more efficiently than creatinine because urea has a lower molecular weight and is therefore more easily cleared.

In the presence of persistent vomiting from any cause more urea than creatinine is lost in the vomitus. Urea diffuses into all body fluids more freely than does creatinine and hence it is more available for loss from the stomach.

The urea/creatinine ratio is also reduced in severe liver failure due to hepatic inability to metabolize amino acids to urea. The actual blood figures would be lower than in this discussion, e.g. urea 2.1 (14 mg/100 ml) and creatinine 148 μmol/1 (1.7 mg/100 ml).

Answer 4.13

These figures were derived from a patient with a GFR of 14 ml/min who was taking a 30 g protein diet. This explains the discrepancy between the urea and creatinine concentrations which would not be found in acute renal failure. In chronic renal failure hypocalcaemia is very frequent. The raised phosphate is found in both conditions. Likewise the serum urate rises in both and is of no discriminatory help. The mild hyperlipidaemia is slight evidence in favour of a chronic lesion as mild elevation of serum lipids is found in many of these patients. The *U/P* ratio of 1.5 implies little concentration but it was measured when there was a normal urine flow rate and such a ratio is compatible with normal renal function under these circumstances. A ratio of 1.1–1.3 in the presence of oliguria (less than 30 ml of urine per hour) would be evidence of acute renal failure. The haemoglobin is only slightly reduced which is against chronic renal disease but there is no direct relationship between nitrogen retention and haemoglobin. In patients with a GFR of more than 20 ml/min only mild anaemia may be present.

Answer 4.14

Haemoglobin: this is low in established chronic renal failure – about 8 g/dl (g/100 ml) or less – and is usually normal in early acute renal failure.

Blood urea: in chronic renal failure in a patient taking a low protein diet urea may be only moderately raised (15–20 mmol/l (90–120 mg/100 ml)) and is also moderately raised in early acute renal failure; therefore it is no help in distinguishing between the two conditions.

Plasma sodium: this is usually not helpful in either case.

Plasma potassium: hyperkalaemia may be present in acute renal failure, but also in some cases of chronic renal failure.

Serum calcium: this electrolyte is usually normal in acute renal failure and is low in established chronic renal failure – about 2.0 mmol/l (8 mg/100 ml).

Serum phosphate: this may be normal or raised in acute renal failure and in established chronic renal failure is regularly raised to about 1.9 mmol/l (6 mg/100 ml) or more.

Answer 4.15

(*a*) The patient had nephrotic syndrome.

(*b*) There had been a rapid decline in renal function with worsening of the nephrotic syndrome. This rate of decline is disproportionate to the expected prognosis of a nephrotic syndrome of any cause. In the presence of sterile urine it is probable that a renal venous thrombosis had occurred. This is an infrequent but recognized complication of nephrotic syndrome of any origin.

(*c*) Selective renal venous catheterization should be performed. If a thrombus is demonstrated intrarenal arterial urokinase infusion should be considered.

Answer 4.16

This man may have had one of three conditions:

(*i*) He may have had no disturbance of carbohydrate metabolism and the previous report of glycosuria was spurious.

(*ii*) He may be a mild diabetic as the shape of a curve plotted from these figures is that of a normal GTT curve, except that at 60 minutes a blood glucose concentration of 9.8 mmol/l (167 mg/100 ml) is high.

(*iii*) He may have renal glycosuria. In this condition some of the nephrons have a lower maximum tubular reabsorption for glucose (Tm_G) than the usual 9.7 mmol/l (175 mg/100 ml) and glycosuria occurs at lower levels of blood glucose concentration.

Answer 4.17

A rise in blood urea of 16.8 mmol/l (101 mg/100 ml) in 24 hours is very rapid. Such a patient will have had pre-existing renal disease. Possible causes include:

(*i*) 'Hypercatabolic' acute renal failure.

(*ii*) Gastrointestinal haemorrhage in a patient with chronic renal failure.

(*iii*) A sharp deterioration in renal function in a patient with chronic renal failure ('acute on chronic' renal failure).

(*iv*) This change may occur in a patient with septicaemia being treated with high dose steroids for a transplant kidney rejection.

(*v*) A laboratory error should also be suspected.

Answer 4.18

This was a spurious hyperkalaemia due to the blood sample having been left too long before centrifugation. Under these conditions red cell potassium leaks into the plasma leading to falsely high readings.

This woman is unlikely to have acute renal failure because hyperkalaemia in these patients is associated with acidosis and the plasma phosphate is very frequently raised. The data do not fit a diagnosis of chronic renal failure because in such people anaemia, hypocalcaemia and hyperphosphataemia are almost invariable. The data would fit the condition of hypoaldosteronism but this is a very rare disease.

Answer 4.19

This patient had a systemic acidosis with acid urine, hypocalcuria and one of the histological features of osteomalacia. The mean width of osteoid borders in undecalcified normal bone is about 9 μm. The osteomalacia and hypocalcuria suggest chronic renal failure. The urine is acid which is almost invariable in chronic renal failure and contrasts with a renal tubular acidosis in which the urine rarely has a pH of below 6.

The differential diagnosis therefore includes renal calcification secondary to hypercalcaemia, renal cortical necrosis or long-standing renal tuberculosis. The first of these conditions is the most common in Britain. The low urine calcium is explained by the renal failure secondary to renal damage consequent upon (previous) hypercalcaemia. When the GFR falls to below 20—25 ml/min hypocalcuria (less than 2.5 mmol/day (100 mg/day)) is virtually constant regardless of the concentration of the serum calcium.

Answer 4.20

(*a*) The presumptive diagnosis is that of an acute transplant rejection as indicated by the high neutrophil count with the reduced lymphocyte count and the low urine volume. In addition, flu-like symptoms are frequently associated with acute graft rejection. Single measurements of creatinine clearance and protein excretion of 4.7 g/24 h do not contribute to the diagnosis unless related to previous measurements. However the development of proteinuria or an increase if already present are features of transplant rejection.

(*b*) Other findings include fever, hypertension, tenderness of the transplanted kidney, increase in urinary lymphocytes, fall in circulating platelets and serum complement components.

Answer 4.21

This man had a hypernephroma as suggested by the haematuria and the abnormal IVP. Raised alkaline phosphatase and abnormal BSP retention are occasionally associated with a hypernephroma in the absence of metastatic spread. This is unexplained. Liver function returns to normal after removal of the renal cancer.

Answer 4.22

(a) There was a very reduced urinary sodium and a high potassium in proportion to that ingested. These are features of hyperaldosteronism and may be found in congestive heart failure, cirrhosis with ascites and nephrotic syndrome.

(b) The urinary urea and creatinine are within the normal range, implying an adequate glomerular filtration rate; this argues against congestive heart failure, in which the GFR is reduced. A very low calcium excretion is a frequent feature of nephrotic syndrome with avid sodium retention. Symmetrically enlarged and smooth kidneys are a very constant finding in nephrotic syndrome. The urinary electrolytes stated in this example are typical of acute nephrotic syndrome.

(c) The urinary excretion of protein should be measured: it would be in the 10–30 g/day range.

Answer 4.23

(a) This patient had established acute renal failure. The U/P ratio for urea is 6.9 and for osmolarity is 1.08. Normally the U/P ratio for urea is 10 or more and the osmolarity U/P ratio is 2–3. If urea and osmolar ratios fall below 10 and 1.1 respectively, established acute renal failure is present. In addition in acute renal failure urine sodium is often more than 70 mmol/l (mEq/l).

(b) It is improbable that this patient would respond to intravenous fluid and an appropriate dose of a loop diuretic (frusemide or bumetamide). In a few patients there might be an increase in water excretion but no increase in concentrating ability of the kidney.

(c) A high dose IVP would very probably show a dense persistent nephrogram which in itself would support the diagnosis of acute renal failure.

Answer 4.24

(a) This man had primary hyperaldosteronism (Conn's syndrome). There was hypertension with low renin and a high plasma aldosterone. The normal response to a low sodium diet is an increase in renin concentration but in the presence of an adrenal adenoma producing aldosterone the response is blocked.

(b) An essential investigation is the measurement of renal venous aldosterone to decide in which adrenal the adenoma is situated.

(c) The condition may be treated with spironalactone which is very effective but expensive and its side effects (gynaecomastia, hirsutes and gastric intolerance) may be limiting in some patients. Definitive treatment is surgical removal of the adenoma after which there is a good chance that the blood pressure will return to normal and remain so.

Answer 4.25

(*a*) The important point to note is that the plasma levels of renin and aldosterone were high after diet A and fell on diet B. Diet A was therefore a low sodium diet – say 10–20 mmol (mEq) per day. As the sodium sensors detected decreased body sodium, renin production was stimulated and hence aldosterone production. This is a normal homeostatic response to a low sodium intake. During the second week dietary sodium was normal or elevated – say 100–200 mmol (mEq) daily. There was therefore need to excrete sodium and the renin–angiotensin–aldosterone axis cut back to allow urinary sodium excretion to rise.

(*b*) During diet A (low sodium) week urinary volume would be proportional to fluid intake, given that no excessive solute load had been taken in the diet. The urinary sodium was less than 10 mmol (mEq) per day. This is the normal renal response to a very low sodium intake. At the end of the second week the urine volume would have risen to excrete the increased sodium load. Again this is a normal renal response.

Answer 4.26

(*a*) This man had many features of a generalized renal tubular defect. There was a tubular type of proteinuria, generalized amino-aciduria and a raised uric acid clearance (normal about 6–8 ml/min) and raised phosphate clearance (implied by the subnormal plasma concentration), impaired ability to acidify the urine, reduced urinary concentrating power and a border-line systemic acidosis. All these features are compatible with the adult Fanconi syndrome.

(*b*) The glycosuria is of the renal type and a standard glucose tolerance test would have a normal or 'flat' curve.

Answer 4.27

(*a*) This woman had a post-abortion haemolytic anaemia with haemaglobulinaemia and bilirubinaemia (black/red urine). The high white blood cell count reflected both the haemolytic anaemia and the presence of infection – most probably due to *Clostridium welchii* as this organism is frequently recovered in patients with septic abortion. *Clostridium welchii* produces a lecithinase which disrupts red blood cells and platelets.

(*b*) Probable complications include: (*i*) septicaemia; (*ii*) disseminated intravascular coagulation (possibly already present; see platelet count); (*iii*) acute renal failure; (*iv*) cortical necrosis; (*v*) death.

Answer 4.28

The differential diagnosis is between pituitary diabetes insipidus and compulsive water drinking. In compulsive water drinking the plasma osmolarity tends to be less than 290 mmol/l and in diabetes insipidus above 290 mmol/l. If a patient with pituitary diabetes insipidus is treated with pitressin the polyuria and thirst cease and the urine osmolarity rises. In patients with compulsive water drinking, pitressin has a much less marked effect as their thirst is not related to polyuria but to their neurotic personalities. Water intoxication may develop in this circumstance.

From the data of this woman the diagnosis was compulsive water drinking.

Answer 4.29

(a) This man had osteomalacia and nephrocalcinosis. These two findings alone are very suggestive of adult (distal) renal tubular acidosis. There was no evidence of malabsorption from the gut in this patient and he had a neutral to only mildly acidic urine in the presence of a systemic acidosis. These findings are entirely compatible with renal tubular acidosis.

(b) The definitive investigation is the demonstration of failure of the urine pH to fall below 5.4 after an acid load – usually given as ammonium chloride 0.1 g/kg bodyweight. In renal tubular acidosis there is an inability to maintain a gradient of hydrogen ions across the distal renal tubule: a persistent acidosis results which impairs maintenance of bone calcification with resulting osteomalacia.

Answer 4.30

From the above figures this subject is normal. Her urinary sodium excretion, plasma renin activity and urinary aldosterone before 9 α-fluorohydrocortisone are all normal and mutually compatible 9 α-fluorohydrocortisone has powerful sodium-retaining properties. This drug over-rides the renin–aldosterone axis and the concentration in these two hormones falls to a low level.

Answer 4.31

These figures are compatible with:

(i) Pregnancy: the GFR and hence the creatinine clearance rises to 40–50% above normal from about the 3rd to 8th month of pregnancy and glycosuria is found in up to 40% of pregnant women as the Tm_G falls.

(*ii*) Nephrotic syndrome: raised creatinine clearance is found in some of these patients due to an increased renal loss of creatinine. In addition glycosuria is found in a proportion of nephrotic patients unrelated to diabetes. The glycosuria is considered to be an expression of tubular dysfunction in this syndrome.

(*iii*) Acromegaly: the GFR and hence the creatinine clearance rises due to increased renal size secondary to growth hormone. In addition diabetes is common in acromegalics.

Answer 4.32

(*a*) A sudden deterioration in renal function associated with haematuria is very suggestive of cancer of the lower urinary tract with bleeding, and obstruction of one or both ureters. This man had lost approximately 75% of his GFR in two months. While renal impairment follows hypertension this is usually found in the patient with accelerated hypertension, and is unusual and gradual in a severe essential hypertensive. In this man's IVP the right kidney with a dilated pelvis suggested a bladder tumour which had previously obstructed the left ureter and had encroached upon the right ureteric orifice.

(*b*) Cystoscopy is essential and showed in this patient an extensive bladder tumour. The left ureteric orifice could not be identified and the right was catheterized with difficulty. Injection of contrast demonstrated a hydro-ureter above the bladder.

(*c*) While hypertension is occasionally a cause of haematuria it is a diagnosis by exclusion. Virtually all middle-aged patients with haematuria require an IVP and cystoscopy regardless of their blood pressure.

Answer 4.33

(*a*) Trace A represents acute obstruction to the upper third of the urinary tract.

(*b*) This was due to a stone in the renal pelvis which was removed (pyelolithotomy).

(*c*) Trace B is the curve obtained from a kidney with normal drainage.

(*d*) The second operation was removal of a parathyroid adenoma.

(*e*) Investigations leading to parathyroid surgery include serum calcium and phosphate, stone analysis, urinary calcium estimation and serum parathormone assay.

NEUROLOGICAL DISEASE

Answer 5.1

(a) It was very probable that this patient had a disseminated sclerosis. An increase in γ-globulin without increase in the total protein content of the CSF is found in about 60% of patients with established disease. This increase in γ-globulin explains the abnormal colloidal gold curve.

(b) In about 20–30% of patients with disseminated sclerosis a high titre of measles antibodies in the CSF is found although the interpretation of this observation is unclear.

Answer 5.2

This patient may have either early poliomyelitis, non-paralytic or paralytic, or the Guillain–Barré syndrome. At an early stage the CSF findings of these two diseases can be very similar and the differentiation is clinical. If CSF were re-examined a week later, that from a poliomyelitis patient would have a pleocytosis and no further increase in protein, while CSF from a patient with Guillain–Barré syndrome would have no pleocytosis but the well recognized increase in protein would be present. CSF culture might later grow the polio virus.

Answer 5.3

(a) The baby was small although the weight gain was adequate for the age assuming that the child was born at term. However the head circumference was disproportionately small.

(b) Microcephaly may be congenital (when it is sometimes familial) or acquired. Transplacentally transmitted infections may be associated with poor head growth. Perinatal asphyxia and bacterial meningitis in early life may interfere with head growth. Metabolic disorders such as phenylketonuria may also be found.

(c) Additional investigations indicated are the following:

(i) Skull X-ray and possible air studies.

(ii) Blood for rubella haemagglutination inhibition, cytomegalovirus and toxoplasma titres.

(iii) Blood and urine amino acid measurements when fasting.

(iv) EEG.

Answer 5.4

A: Anterior cerebral artery. Obstruction leads to a spastic monoplegia with or without cortical loss of the sensory type. There may be a grasp reflex of the opposite upper limb and apraxia if the left anterior cerebral artery is affected.

B: Middle cerebral artery. Occlusion results in hemiplegia, crossed homonymous hemianopia, loss of spatial and discriminative sensibility on the opposite side of the body and aphasia if the lesion is on the left side.

C: Posterior cerebral artery. Occlusion is followed by a crossed homonymous hemianopia. The macula may be spared.

D: Basilar artery. Thrombosis of this vessel is usually rapidly fatal preceded by loss of consciousness, small fixed pupils and quadriplegia.

E: Posterior inferior cerebellar artery. At the onset of occlusion there is vertigo, dysphagia and at times pain or parathesiae over the Vth ipsilateral cranial nerve. Cerebellar signs are present and an ipsilateral Horner's syndrome. There is analgesia of the face on the same side as the lesion and of the trunk and limbs on the opposite side.

Answer 5.5

(*a*) Cushing's disease due to a pituitary chromophobe or basophil adenoma producing an excess of ACTH.

(*b*) Removal of the adrenal glands removes the site of excess cortisol production but not the primary cause. The pituitary continues to produce an excess of ACTH (normal range about 15–80 pg/ml) and β-MSH. The β-MSH excess leads to excess pigmentation and in this context the clinical picture is referred to as Nelson's syndrome.

(*c*) In the patient under discussion the visual impairment is likely to be due to compression of the optic chiasm by the upward expansion of the pituitary tumour first compressing the decussating fibres and giving rise to bitemporal hemianopia. Treatment would probably involve surgical removal of the tumour.

Answer 5.6

(*a*) This boy had Wilson's disease. The serum copper is in the normal range (80–140 μg/100 ml) and in patients with Wilson's disease the range is 10–110 μg/100 ml. A proportion of these patients go through a self-limiting phase of a Coombs' negative haemolytic anaemia with subclinical hepatic disease and subsequently present with neurological, psychiatric or renal tubular disease (amino-aciduria, glycosuria and increased clearance of urate). The urine copper in this boy was characteristically raised, the normal range being 5–25 μg/24 h.

(*b*) The serum ceruloplasmin should be measured and would be found to be less than 20 mg/100 ml when the normal range is 25–40 mg/100 ml.

(*c*) The additional sign which is always present when the condition has progressed to the neurological stage is the Kayser–Fleischer ring located at the periphery of the cornea in Descemet's membrane.

Answer 5.7

(*a*) There were two diagnoses. Assuming the blood sample assayed for acid phosphatase was not haemolyzed the concentration of this enzyme is in the range associated with metastatic deposits from carcinoma of the prostate. Also elevated and ranked in ascending order of diagnostic importance are serum alanine transaminase, lactic dehydrogenase and creatinine kinase. All these enzymes tend to be elevated in polymyositis. Often in polymyositis related to a malignancy the muscle disorder becomes apparent before the tumour is demonstratable. Of polymyositis in general an underlying tumour is found in about 10–20% of patients.

(*b*) Electromyography (EMG) of an affected muscle is indicated and will establish the diagnosis with certainty. The features expected to be found are the following:

(*i*) Spontaneous fibrillation.

(*ii*) Salvos of repetitive potentials.

(*iii*) Short duration of polyphasic potentials of low amplitude.

Answer 5.8

A: This is the anterior spinothalamic tract (corticospinal). Fibres concerned with the appreciation of pain, heat and cold ascend in this tract; as similar fibres run in the lateral spinothalamic tract no symptoms may occur if the anterior spinothalamic tract alone is distroyed.

B: This is the lateral spinothalamic tract. No symptoms may occur unless the anterior spinothalamic tract is also distroyed for reasons given above.

C: This is the central canal. A lesion at this site leads to 'disassociated sensory loss' in which appreciation of pain, heat and cold is lost bilaterally over the dermatomes, sensory fibres from which are decussating at the level of the lesion.

D: This is the posterior sensory root. A lesion will thus affect all modalities of sensation.

E: This is the posterior column. A lesion produces abolition of kinaesthesia and serious impairment of touch.

Answer 5.9

(*a*) The occipital–frontal circumference was well above the average for a baby of average head circumference and birth weight.

(*b*) This could be due to congenital hydrocephalus, acquired hydrocephalus secondary to purulent meningitis, hydrocephalus due to tumour of the fourth ventricle, subdural haematoma or porencephaly.

(*c*) Clinical features include: a large full fontanelle, prominent scalp veins and forehead, sunsetting eyes, transillumination of the head, and retarded development status of the child depending on the cause.

(*d*) Additional investigations should include: skull X-ray, subdural and ventricular taps and an air ventriculogram.

Answer 5.10

The head circumference is normal for this age of child. Intracranial calcification could be due to: (*i*) toxoplasmosis; (*ii*) hyperparathyroidism; (*iii*) tuberose sclerosis; (*iv*) Sturge–Weber syndrome.

Answer 5.11

(*a*) α-Fetoprotein in serum is raised in many cases of neural tube defect (spina bifida or ancephaly). A more significant correlation exists between amniotic fluid levels of α-fetoprotein and such defects. The levels rise as pregnancy progresses and more definite results would be obtained at 16–18 weeks than at 11–12 weeks.

(*b*) A raised serum α-fetoprotein should be followed by ultrasound localization of the placenta and amniocentesis. A significantly raised amniotic α-fetoprotein makes a neural tube defect very likely and termination of the pregnancy should be offered. The highest correlation is found between α-fetoprotein and ancephaly. A meningocele may exist with little or no increase in α-fetoprotein. The incidence of neural tube defects is 1:600 in London and 1:250 in South Wales. Where a woman has already had an affected baby the risk rises to 1:40. Serum α-fetoprotein as a screening procedure should therefore become part of routine antenatal care.

(*c*) The other main cause of raised α-fetoprotein is primary hepatoma.

Answer 5.12

This patient most probably had a viral meningitis but very similar CSF findings are found in secondary syphilis although in syphilis the cell count is unlikely to be quite so high as quoted in this example. A rash may be found in both conditions. Syphilitic meningitis is uncommon although abnormal CSF findings are found in 50% of patients with untreated secondary syphilis.

Answer 5.13

(a) This is a typical EEG of *petit mal*.
(b) The temporary 'absences' of *petit mal* might be observed during the EEG recording but the EEG disturbance is not invariably accompanied by clinical manifestations.

Answer 5.14

(a) This patient had cerebral lupus. The high DNA binding (normal less than 30%) indicates a high titre of antibodies against double-stranded DNA. The low C3 suggests complement consumption implying active systemic lupus erythematosis (SLE). The lymphocytopenia is frequently found in active lupus and very frequently in cerebral lupus. There are no characteristic features of the EEG in this condition particularly in the absence of any focal sign. A neurosis is the most common expression of cerebral lupus.
(b) Opinions differ regarding treatment. If there is no clinical evidence of disease elsewhere the patient may only require sedation during the neurotic phase. Other physicians would use steroids with sedatives. If there were focal neurological disease then steroids would be essential.

Answer 5.15

(a) This child had bacterial meningitis as shown by the increased CSF white blood cell count (normal CSF contains less than 3 cells/mm^3), the high neutrophil count, the raised protein (normal 0.15–0.4 g/l (15–40 mg/100 ml)) and lowered glucose concentration.
(b) The immediate immunoglobulin response is of the IgM class.
(c) Gram-staining of the CSF may show intracellular diplococci (meningococci or pneumococci) or Gram-negative rods (*H. influenzae*). A CSF with this high white count would be obviously abnormal as it is withdrawn from the patient.

(*d*) Intrathecal penicillin (about 5000 units for a child aged 13 months) should be given together with intravenous penicillin. Some authorities recommend the immediate use of chloramphenicol and sulphadimidine as well as penicillin at least until the organism is known. High dose ampicillin is also quite widely used in bacterial meningitis.

Answer 5.16

(*a*) This woman had the Ramsey—Hunt syndrome (Herpes zoster of the geniculate ganglion).
(*b*) As the soft palate and external auditory meatus were involved the cutaneous branches of vagus which communicate with the seventh nerve were also affected.
(*c*) Further investigations are needed in view of the very high ESR, the roleaux on the blood film and the hypergammaglobulinaemia. These hint at myeloma. Skull, vertebrae and pelvis should be X-rayed, urine tested for Bence-Jones proteinuria and the bone marrow examined.

Answer 5.17

(*a*) The high CSF protein, mixed cellular response and low glucose in an illness developing over 10 days are suggestive of tuberculous meningitis. High CSF protein and low glucose concentrations are only infrequently found in viral meningitis and the cellular response is typically predominantly lymphocytic. The onset of viral and of bacterial meningitis is much more rapid than in this example.
(*b*) There are three other investigations needed: Z—N staining of the CSF, the setting up of Lowenstein—Jensen cultures and a chest X-ray. In an adult, cytological examination of the CSF is necessary because carcinomatous meningitis has a chronic deteriorating course together with a mixed pleocytosis and reduction in the CSF glucose.

Answer 5.18

(*a*) Hypocalcaemia is the likely cause of the convulsion. In practice such a baby would probably be bottle fed and the phosphate load from the cow's milk formula might well depress the ionized calcium although the total calcium quoted in this example is not particularly low. Hypocalcaemic convulsions do not occur in the breast fed baby and do not arise in the bottle fed until the baby has been receiving milk for several days. Hypoglycaemia is a significant and treatable cause of convulsions in a low birth weight baby as quoted but a blood glucose concentration of 1.7 mmol/1 (30 mg/100 ml) is not of the order to be symptomatic and the child would probably present earlier.

(b) A lumbar puncture would be a necessary investigation – neonatal meningitis must be excluded. Intercranial bleeding in association with haemorrhagic disease of the newborn and/or perinatal asphyxia are possibilities.

Answer 5.19

These data show heart failure and motor neuropathy. Normally conduction of velocity in the fastest fibres is about 60 m/s. The differential diagnosis includes the following:

(i) Diabetic heart failure due to ischaemic heart disease and neuropathy; the latter is usually predominantly sensory.

(ii) Amyloid.

(iii) Myxoedema.

(iv) Beri-beri.

Answer 5.20

(a) These findings are typical Froin's syndrome. Apart from a much raised protein content the CSF pressure failed to vary with the respiration or jugular compression. The commonest cause of this syndrome is an advanced spinal tumour or an area of spinal meningitis.

(b) The differential diagnosis is that of raised CSF protein which at this high concentration includes the Guillain–Barré syndrome and some intercranial tumours especially an acoustic neuroma. The CSF protein is very high at the onset of symptoms in spinal block due to tumour of the cord, whereas in Guillain–Barré syndrome it may be only a little raised at the onset but continues to rise even though the symptoms begin to remit.

METABOLIC CONDITIONS

Answer 6.1

(*a*) It is unlikely that a blood urea of 29 mmol/l (175 mg/100 ml) will produce persistent vomiting; a serum calcium of 3.8 mmol/l (13.5 mg/ 100 ml) is much more likely to be the cause.

(*b*) This case revolves around the hypercalcaemia and primary hyper-parathyroidism could explain all the abnormalities. Hypercalcaemia leads to renal functional impairment (hypercalcaemic nephropathy) which secondarily leads to phosphate retention. However the blood urea is high for such a diagnosis, and one should consider a condition which may cause both hypercalcaemia and renal damage. Myeloma leads to hypercalcaemia via bone lesions and can depress renal function in a number of ways. Theoretically sarcoid may cause both hyper-calcaemia and depression of kidney function but renal sarcoid is rare. A 'myeloma kidney' is relatively common.

Answer 6.2

The most likely explanation of hyponatraemia, hypokalaemia and hypercalcaemia would be an oat cell tumour of a bronchus producing both atopic ADH and parathormone. Many other tumours also have this potential ability. For discussion of ADH effects *see* Answer 6.32, page 150. It should be noted that oat cell tumours tend to produce ADH and squamous cell tumours secreted mainly PTH but there is not an absolute distinction between them.

Answer 6.3

(*i*) This could be *nephrotic syndrome* presenting with a precipitating infection. However, the facial swelling would not be confined to the lower face and proteinuria would probably be more marked. The patient is rather young for this diagnosis.

(*ii*) The patient is again rather young for *mumps* but it is possible at this age. The white cell count and the high neutrophil count are both high for viral infection.

(*iii*) *Osteomyelitis of the jaw* would be a probability. The swelling probably would not be symmetrical and the X-ray is normal initially, changes developing later. Blood culture would be essential; if nega-tive, antistaphylococcal antibody titres would be required.

(*iv*) The X-ray appearances of the jaw are diagnostic of *infantile cortical hyperostosis*. Also changes may well be seen in the ribs when a chest X-ray is taken. Fever, anaemia, lymphocytosis and raised ESR are all compatible with this diagnosis and all become normal with passage of time. The cause is unknown.

Answer 6.4

(*a*) This man was hypocalcaemic with a raised alkaline phosphatase. These findings in this context suggest an inadequate diet and osteomalacia secondary to vitamin D deficiency.

(*b*) X-ray of the vertebrae of this man showed the psuedo-fractures of the scapulae and pubic rami.

(*c*) Treatment involves vitamin D and provision of an adequate diet at home.

Answer 6.5

(*i*) Addison's disease may present with hypoglycaemia and hyponatraemia is the rule.

(*ii*) Advanced liver failure. Hyponatraemia occurs in this condition. The liver fails to clear the normal amount of insulin before it reaches the systemic circulation, giving rise to hypoglycaemia.

(*iii*) Emergency treatment of hyperglycaemia with too much insulin and too little normal saline will cause hypoglycaemia and hyponatraemia.

(*iv*) An oat cell tumour of the bronchus producing inappropriate ADH secretion and insulin activity may occasionally produce findings of this nature.

Answer 6.6

(*a*) Back disease associated with HLA B27 is very suggestive of ankylosing spondylitis. Of patients with ankylosing spondylitis 85% have B27. The prevalence of this antigen in healthy Londoners is about 14%.

(*b*) X-ray of the spine would show the 'bamboo changes' (calcification of the paraspinus ligaments with squaring of the vertebral bodies) and fusion of the sacroiliac joints with surrounding osteosclerosis and osteoporosis.

(*c*) Patients with ankylosing spondylitis have a predisposition to the development of aortic incompetence. The pulse pressure would therefore be increased as some of the left ventricular stroke volume returns to the left ventricle across the incompetent valve.

Answer 6.7

(*i*) Congestive cardiac failure.
(*ii*) Nephrotic syndrome.
(*iii*) Ascites.

The data show: reduced blood volume (normal for males 69 mg/kg bodyweight), raised renin and raised plasma aldosterone. Together these changes constitute secondary hyperaldosteronism which may occur in the above three conditions. Raised plasma aldosterone might suggest Conn's syndrome (primary hyperaldosteronism) but the raised renin and reduced blood volume are not found in this condition. In secondary hyperaldosteronism, arterial hypovolaemia is considered to be the stimulus to renin production. Despite venous congestion in congestive heart failure, arterial hypovolaemia results from the falling cardiac output. Arterial volume may also be diminished due to hypo-albuminaemia resulting from proteinuria in nephrotic syndrome or from deficient albumin synthesis in cirrhosis.

Answer 6.8

No. The calculated osmolarity is 318.4, based on the formula:

$2(Na^+) + 2(K^+) + urea + glucose$
Thus: $300 + 8 + 7.2 + 5.2 = 318.4$ (All concentrations expressed in SI units)

In this example either direct measurement of the plasma osmolarity is incorrect or the plasma sodium (which contributes chiefly to the plasma osmolarity) measurement is inaccurate. The above calculation is not valid if there is gross lipaemia or hyperproteinaemia or following an infusion of mannitol.

Answer 6.9

The abnormalities are hypo-albuminaemia, hyperlipidaemia and raised serum urate.

With hypo-albuminaemia, hyperlipidaemia is common. Usually plasma calcium also falls as there are fewer binding sites for the non-ionized fraction. In this instance the calcium is normal. Renal function judged by plasma creatinine was normal so the raised urate was not the result of a reduced GFR. Insufficient information is given to make a composite diagnosis in this man but the calcium 'raised' relative to the albumin suggests either hyperparathyroidism or excess calcium loss from bones. An occasional patient with malignant bone disease (such as myeloma) may have renal damage causing hypo-albuminaemia and relative or absolute hypercalcaemia. This was the explanation in this patient.

The raised serum urate was an incidental finding: urate rises in myeloma patients following treatment or if there is renal damage.

Answer 6.10

In this question the blood urea was raised while the plasma creatinine was normal. (*i*) The commonest cause is a heavy protein load which occurs after a gut haemorrhage. (*ii*) With a very high protein diet a similar difference between urea and creatinine may be found. (*iii*) Large doses of steroids exert a catabolic effect and hence cause isolated urea elevation. (*iv*) A similar difference between urea and creatinine may occur in a bilateral amputee with about 60% loss of GFR. In this circumstance the amount of creatinine formed is reduced as the body muscle mass is diminished. As there is renal impairment blood concentration of urea and creatinine rise but on a normal diet the urea rises more than the creatinine. (*v*) In the elderly the GFR falls to about 50% of its value in youth due to senile nephron loss. Muscle mass is also reduced in old age. Therefore there is less creatinine produced. The blood urea rises due to the reduced GFR and the creatinine remains in the normal range.

Answer 6.11

(*a*) This man had a high serum iron and an almost fully saturated iron binding capacity. He was diabetic and had a raised SGPT. This man had idiopathic haemochromatosis. There is almost no differential diagnosis from these findings. Transfusion haemosiderosis is excluded as the patient was previously well and haemosiderosis from prolonged iron therapy is very uncommon.

(*b*) The fully established clinical picture of haemochromatosis is a combination of liver disease, diabetes, heart disease and skin pigmentation. There is an increased chance of a primary hepatoma. There are therefore many possible clinical features of this condition. Men are very much more frequently affected than women.

Answer 6.12

(a) This patient had Type A lactic acidosis, that is, lactic acidosis and tissue anoxia (Type B is lactic acidosis without tissue anoxia).

(b) and (c) Type A is found in association with cardiogenic shock, endotoxaemia, left ventricular failure and very severe anaemias. The mortality may be up to 100%. Type B lactic acidosis is subdivided into two groups (Cohen and Woods, 1976)*:

(i)   In association with diabetes mellitus, liver failure, renal failure and leukaemias.
(ii) Related to drugs especially biguanides (phenformin and metformin) and parenteral nutrition with fructose, sorbitol, zylitol or ethanol. An overdose of methanol or salicylates also causes lactic acidosis.

(d) Treatment involves correction of the underlying condition and administration of intravenous bicarbonate of which very large quantities may be required.

Answer 6.13

This man had pyrophosphate arthropathy (pseudogout, chondro-calcinosis). While features of this man's investigations suggest gout, the weakly positive birefringence of the joint crystals makes the diagnosis of pseudogout. Joint crystals of uric acid have a strong negative birefringence while those of calcium pyrophosphate dihydrate possess weak positive birefringence. The serum urate in this man was only about the upper limit of normal for his age although compatible with the diagnosis of gout.

Answer 6.14

(a) The patient was unconscious and the blood glucose by calculation from the plasma osmolarity, sodium, potassium and urea was 29.3 mmol/l (527 mg/100 ml). (For details of the calculation see Answer 6.8, page 142). A blood glucose of this severity is one cause for the coma.

*Cohen, R. D. and Woods, H. F. (1976). *Clinical and Biochemical Aspects of Lactic Acidosis.* Oxford; Blackwell Scientific

(b) The 6 week history of headache in an Asian immigrant together with high CSF protein make the diagnosis of tuberculous meningitis a serious possibility. Ziehl–Neelsen staining of the CSF confirmed the diagnosis.

(c) The very high serum osmolarity is due to the high concentration of glucose and the hypernatraemia. The high urine osmolarity superficially is surprising in the presence of the raised blood urea. However the raised urea is simply a measure of dehydration consequent upon an osmotic diuresis and the diuretic, glucose, produces the raised urinary osmolarity.

Answer 6.15

No diagnosis is possible from these figures. The man did not have gout as the uric acid is not in the pathological range for a male aged 72 years. Likewise the blood urea is normal for the age. The normal ESR is a further point against an acute inflammatory joint lesion. The ANF was of low titre and is not infrequently found in elderly patients – it has no diagnostic significance. A probable cause of this man's symptom would be degenerative joint disease.

Answer 6.16

(a) This is Frederickson's Type III hyperlipoproteinaemia. All the biochemical features of this condition, which is usually inherited, are mentioned in the question.

(b) It is usually associated with cardiovascular disease including peripheral vascular disease, xanthomata, impaired carbohydrate tolerance and hyperuricaemia.

(c) Type III hyperlipoproteinaemia responds well to clofibrate and cholestyramine. Restriction of dietary cholesterol and saturated fats is also usually recommended.

Answer 6.17

(a) The birth weight was low for a term baby. Causes of dismaturity include transplacentally acquired infections: rubella, toxoplasmosis and cytomegalovirus inclusion disease. Any of these conditions can give rise to a form of hepatitis – hence the jaundice and prolonged prothrombin time. In the case of rubella syndrome thrombocytopenia may contribute to a tendency to bleed.

The weight loss was more than 10% of the birth weight and was therefore more than a physiological degree of weight loss. This may be a feature of all of the above but it is also seen in postnatally acquired bacterial infections and in galactosaemia. Bleeding and jaundice occur in galactosaemia also.

(b) Further investigations would include: cytomegalovirus and rubella titres and toxoplasma complement fixation tests. Urine should be examined for reducing substances and if positive red cell galactose-l-phospholate-uridyl-transferase should be assayed.

Answer 6.18

(a) This woman had osteoporosis as shown by the normal serum calcium and phosphate and the normal urinary calcium. The raised alkaline phosphatase in this patient was a reflection upon the fracture and fell to normal when the bone healed.

(b) Confirmation of the diagnosis usually rests upon radiological thinning and reduction in the trabecular pattern of bones, the femoral necks and vertebrae being the best areas to show these features. Bone densitometry and bone biopsy may also be used.

(c) Osteoporosis may be secondary to: (i) partial gastrectomy; (ii) other causes of malabsorption; (iii) Cushing's syndrome; (iv) hyperthyroidism; (v) liver disease; (vi) hypogonadism; (vii) scurvy.

Answer 6.19

The further investigations include thyroid function tests, growth hormone estimation and the exclusion of malabsorption. The bone age may be retarded to some extent in many causes of growth retardation. Where physical examination is normal and the child appears in good health congenital hypothyroidism is unlikely but juvenile myxoedema may occur and the diagnosis should be considered. Thyroxine and thyroid-stimulating hormone should be measured. A low TSH implies a pituitary lesion which may be further elucidated by a TRH stimulation test. Similarly, malabsorption is unlikely in an apparently healthy child but symptoms should be sought in the history.

Growth hormone estimation is necessary. Growth hormone deficiency is commoner in males and a child may well grow normally initially, presenting in the third or fourth year of life as the growth weight falls off. A normal birth weight is usual in these patients. Growth hormone deficiency is usually an isolated defect but may be part of a general hypopituitarism.

146

Answer 6.20

The clue to this question is that the blood was obtained with 'some difficulty'. The figures show respiratory alkalosis but this may have been induced via hyperventilation because of pain at the time of arterial puncture. Unless the patient has cause for a respiratory alkalosis the blood gas data should be interpreted with care.

Answer 6.21

(a) The anion gap is calculated from the formula $(Na + K) - (Cl + HCO_3)$. Therefore $(142 + 5) - (104 + 25) = 18$.

(b) The gap represents approximately the sum of the unmeasured anions (protein, sulphate, phosphate, lactate and 3-hydroxybutyrate) the charges of which must, together with those of chloride and bicarbonate, balance those of the cations sodium and potassium. As charge is involved the constituents must be expressed in mEq/l and not mmol/l.

(c) The major causes of an increased gap are metabolic acidosis, severe renal failure, ketoacidosis, the acidotic phase of salicylate poisoning and lactic acidosis. Less common causes of metabolic acidosis include methanol and ethylene glycol poisoning.

It should be noted that a metabolic acidosis can occur in the presence of a normal anion gap. This is found when chloride has replaced bicarbonate as in renal tubular acidosis, ureterosigmoidostomy and in bicarbonate loss in severe persistent diarrhoea.

Answer 6.22

The most likely diagnosis is eclampsia. The explanation is as follows: proteinuria of 3.4 g/day is insufficient to cause hypo-albuminaemic oedema. The serum urate is raised in eclampsia and is disproportionately high for a creatinine clearance of 78 ml/min due to primary renal causes. Hypertension, oedema and convulsions are the triad that comprises eclampsia. Lactosuria is frequent in pregnant women.

Answer 6.23

(a) This boy was an example of the rare Lesch–Nyhan syndrome. The combination of the neurological features and the excessively raised serum urate makes the diagnosis.

(*b*) The disease is a sex-linked recessive inborn error of metabolism in which there is a lack of the enzyme hypoxanthine-guanine phosphoriposyl transferase (Hg-PRTase). This enzyme catalyses the conversion of hypoxanthine and guanine to their respective nucleotides — inosinic acid and guanylic acid. In the absence of Hg-PRTase an excess of hypoxanthine and xanthine develops which is metabolized to urate by xanthine oxidase. It is thought that the features of the Lesch—Nyhan syndrome result in increased concentrations of hypoxanthine and guanine in those tissues which normally contain Hg-PRTase. The brain and basal ganglia in particular are affected.

Answer 6.24

This patient had all the clinical features of Marfan's syndrome. In those patients in whom dislocation of the lens occurs it is important to test for homocystinuria (cystathionine synthetase deficiency) as many patients with homocystinuria have the same body configuration as in Marfan's syndrome.

Answer 6.25

(*a*) It is generally agreed that patients with primary gout have an increased incidence of Type IV hyperlipoproteinaemia.
(*b*) The plasma in Type IV hyperlipoproteinaemia is turbid due to a raised triglyceride concentration of about 2—10 mmol/l (175—885 mg/ 100 ml) and at times with cholesterol elevation. There is an increase in the pre-β-lipoproteins.

Answer 6.26

The first point to notice is the systemic alkalosis associated with a raised urea. If this urea were a reflection upon renal parenchymal damage the bicarbonate would be in the normal range. The next step is to calculate the plasma chloride: $(Na + K) - (HCO_3 + Cl)$ = anion gap. Therefore $Cl = 138 - 44 = 94$. This patient was therefore depleted of sodium, chloride and potassium. These features together with the alkalosis are typical of persistent vomiting due to pyloric stenosis.

Sodium and potassium are lost in the vomitus but proportionately more hydrogen and chloride ions are lost. Gastric juice contains approximately sodium 50, chloride 45, potassium 12 and hydrogen 50 mmol/l.

The renal response to persistent vomiting is to conserve sodium at the expense of potassium and hydrogen ions. Because of the loss of hydrogen ions from the stomach alkalosis develops and this effect is additive to the renal exchange of potassium and hydrogen ions for sodium ions.

(b) The urine is likely to be acid despite the systemic alkalosis.

Answer 6.27

A: Normal.

B: Uncompensated respiratory alkalosis as in hyperventilation.

C: Uncompensated respiratory acidosis as in acute and chronic chest diseases.

D: Combination of non-respiratory alkalosis and a respiratory acidosis. This represents compensation of the respiratory acidosis.

E: Uncompensated non-respiratory acidosis as seen in aspirin overdose, diabetic ketoacidosis, advanced renal failure and lactic acidosis. In the presence of a non-respiratory acidosis renal compensation is less efficient than in the presence of a respiratory acidosis because hydrogen ion excretion increases with a raised P_{CO_2} and P_{CO_2} will be within normal limits in a non-respiratory acidosis. The distal tubules of the kidney generate more ammonia which combines with the hydrogen ions in the tubular fluid partially correcting the acidosis. Given a steady rate of hydrogen ion production leading to a non-respiratory acidosis and subsequent renal compensation, arterial pH will rise to 7.35–7.4 but the plasma bicarbonate will remain at about 12–15 mmol/l (mEq/l).

F: Non-respiratory and respiratory acidosis. Renal compensation is better than in example E for reasons given above. In addition the increased renal hydrogen ion excretion allows absorption of bicarbonate from renal tubular fluid. This explains the bicarbonate of 20 mmol/l (mEq/l).

Answer 6.28

(a) This patient was hypocalcaemic, hypophosphataemic and had a very low level of 25-OHD$_3$ (the immediate metabolite of vitamin D$_3$). This was vitamin D deficiency either of dietary origin or secondary to severe malabsorption. The patient will have rickets if a child or osteomalacia if an adult.

(b) Symptoms will be of bone pain, expressed in general misery in small children, related to abnormal bone metabolism. Clinical bone deformity may be demonstrable.

Answer 6.29

This is a flat GTT curve and it is found in four groups of people:

(*i*) Patients with malabsorption. However, a flat GTT is not by itself diagnostic of malabsorption.
(*ii*) Patients with untreated Addison's disease — after replacement therapy the curve becomes normal.
(*iii*) In people with growth hormone deficiency. The absence of growth hormone enhances muscle uptake of glucose.
(*iv*) In otherwise normal people. This observation is unexplained.

Answer 6.30

There are only two possibilities: either there was an error in measuring the electrolytes or the blood taken for these investigations had been inadvertently diluted. Such a dilution occurs if the venous blood sample is taken from the same vein into which dextrose is being infused.

Answer 6.31

(*a*) These are the biochemical findings of a phaeochromocytoma. The blood sugar, serum potassium, plasma noradrenaline, urinary meta-nephrines and 4-hydroxy-3-methoxy mandelic acid (HMMA) are all elevated. The excretion products of catecholamines and raised plasma noradrenaline are also found after clonidine withdrawal. Raised HMMA may be found in patients taking reserpine, guanethidine, α-methyldopa and phenothiazines because excretion products of these drugs interfere with the assay of HMMA.
(*b*) There is no drug which will reverse the biochemical features of a secreting phaeochromocytoma. The blood pressure can be controlled by alpha blockade but the production of catecholamines is unaffected.

Answer 6.32

This was hyponatraemia in the presence of normal renal function. There are three conditions in which this electrolyte picture is found:

(*i*) Intravenous infusion for a few days after abdominal surgery with dextrose or dextrose saline (0.18% sodium chloride). Effectively this is infusing only water and the patient becomes sodium depleted.

There is a tendency for the blood urea to be elevated. This is the most common cause.

(*ii*) In appropriate ADH secretion. This is much less common. The hyponatraemia is dilutional due to water retention. One of the most common causes in Western Europe is an anaplastic tumour of the bronchus.

(*iii*) Spurious hyponatraemia is occasionally found in the presence of severe hyperlipidaemia or hyperproteinaemia. These are rare conditions.

Answer 6.33

(*a*) This woman had either primary (Conn's syndrome) or secondary hyperaldosteronism. Hypokalaemia, alkalosis and raised excretion of aldosterone are features of both.

(*b*) The differentiation between these two conditions is simple: hypotensive therapy is withdrawn for a period of 2–3 weeks and the patient is then reinvestigated. If there were primary hyperaldosteronism the plasma and urinary findings would be unchanged. If hyperaldosteronism had developed secondary to the diuretic treatment the abnormal biochemical features would revert to normal after therapy had been withdrawn.

Answer 6.34

(*a*) This woman had an iron deficiency anaemia, hypercalcaemia, hypermagnesaemia with a low serum phosphate, hypercalcuria and an infected urine. The simplest explanation of these findings is primary hyperparathyroidism (raised serum and urine calcium and low serum phosphate) complicated by (*i*) the development of a duodenal ulcer which had led to the development of an iron deficiency anaemia; (*ii*) the development of a renal stone — haematuria and an *E. Coli* infection. The elevated calcium and depressed phosphate are very characteristic of primary hyperparathyroidism. Hypermagnesaemia is found in a proportion of these patients and returns to normal with removal of the parathyroid adenoma.

(*b*) Radiologically an IVP and barium meal are indicated and in that order so that no barium remains in the gut to obscure X-rays of the renal tract.

(*c*) The primary abnormality can be confirmed by measurement of circulating parathyroid hormone (PTH) although from the above data it would not be necessary.

Answer 6.35

(*a*) Severe backache and abnormalities of micturition in an elderly man suggest carcinoma of the prostate with metastases to vertebrae. In this patient the acid phosphatase was raised as is the rule with secondary forms of this neoplasm. The raised alkaline phosphatase reflected bone osteoblastic activity around the site of the metastases.

(*b*) The bone origin of the alkaline phosphatase could be confirmed by electrophoresis of the enzyme. The prostatic carcinoma should be confirmed by prostatic biopsy and the vertebral disease by X-ray which will show sclerotic areas corresponding to the metastases.

Answer 6.36

(*a*) (*i*) Hypernatraemia secondary to gastroenteritis; (*ii*) renal insufficiency precipitated by infection on the basis of congenitally abnormal kidneys; (*iii*) adrenogenital syndrome; (*iv*) transient neonatal hyperglycaemia; (*v*) nephrogenic diabetes insipidus.

(*b*) Additional investigations include urine sample for microscopy and culture, stool culture, blood culture, blood glucose measurement, urine collection for assay of 17-ketosteroids, 17-hydroxycorticosteroids, and IVP.

The likely cause is infection of the gastrointestinal tract. Persistence in feeding milk to a baby with diarrhoea and vomiting may lead to elevation of the plasma sodium since fluid loss is disproportionate to solute loss. Renal reserve in the infant is limited and a rise in urea and a fall in bicarbonate may rapidly occur.

Diarrhoea may be a non-specific symptom and the infection should be looked for in other areas — urine and blood particularly. If the infection is in the urinary tract an underlying congenital abnormality of the renal tract should be subsequently excluded.

If the dehydration appears disproportionate to the proceeding symptoms, underlying metabolic disorders should be considered. Adrenogenital syndrome may present in this way. Virilization in the male may not be apparent at this early age. Patients with the commonest type — 21 hydroxylase deficiency — are however salt losers. Urinary pregnanediol, gonadotrophins and 17-ketosteroids are elevated.

Nephrogenic diabetes insipidus is a sex-linked disorder and may present in early life. Gross elevation of blood glucose with hyperosmolar dehydration is found in transient neonatal diabetes mellitus — which is rare.

Answer 6.37

There was a hypokalaemic alkalosis in the presence of normal renal function. There are six widely recognized causes:

(*i*)   Long-term diuretic therapy; this is the commonest cause.

(*ii*) Corticosteroid therapy: the sodium-retaining properties of the steroid causes secondary renal potassium loss.

(*iii*) Cushing's disease: the same mechanism operates as in (*ii*).

(*iv*) Conn's syndrome: aldosterone excess causes sodium retention with secondary potassium loss whether from an adrenal adenoma or bilateral adrenal hyperplasia.

(*v*)   Excess dosage of carbenoxolone sodium in the treatment of gastric ulcer. Carbenoxolone has a renal potassium excretory effect as has liquorice, which is also used in the treatment of ulcer.

(*vi*) Purgative abuse. Potassium is the major ion of the large bowel; excess purgation leads to potassium depletion.

Answer 6.38

(*a*) This woman had gout. The combination of a very painful joint with a raised serum urate made the diagnosis.

(*b*) Confirmation of the diagnosis would be by demonstration of crystals of uric acid in fluid aspirated from the joint. Therapeutic confirmation would be obtained with colchicine therapy which will control the pain within hours.

(*c*) This attack of gout was pecipitated by the thiazide diuretic taken to control the heart failure. All thiazide diuretics tend to decrease urinary urate excretion although the mechanism is unknown.

Answer 6.39

(*a*) This infant had Bartter's syndrome.

(*b*) A renal biopsy would show marked hypertrophy of the juxtaglomerular apparatus.

(*c*) The cause of the condition was considered to be a diminished ability of the proximal tubule to reabsorb sodium leading to excess sodium reaching the distal tubule. The sodium and water loss reduces the extracellular fluid volume leading to a fall in blood pressure and raised renin, angiotensin and aldosterone. Subsequently it has been found that prostaglandin production (at least by the kidney) is much increased and if this is blocked by a drug such as indomethacin which inhibits prostaglandin synthetase virtually all parameters of the condition return to normal. The success of indomethacin in this condition makes the aetiology more obscure.

Answer 6.40

(*a*) There was haemodilution, hyperkalaemia and respiratory acidosis. The haemodilution is consequent upon the inhalation and absorption of water across the alveoli. This is characteristic of fresh water drowning. Respiratory acidosis occurs following inhalation of either fresh or salt water. Hyperkalaemia is a feature of both. Therefore this man died of fresh water drowning.

(*b*) Immediately before a fresh water death ventricular fibrillation is the usual arrhythmia; after sea water, asystole.

HAEMATOLOGY

Answer 7.1

This woman had a low serum iron in the presence of a normal marrow appearance. This is a common but non-specific finding in ill people. It is seen in a variety of diseases as part of a response to 'inflammation' without any concomitant iron deficiency. An additional but probably not clinically important point is that the blood sample was taken towards the end of day. Serum iron has a diurnal variation, being higher in the morning than the evening.

Answer 7.2

(*a*) This woman had paroxysmal nocturnal haemoglobinuria.

(*b*) Blood and urine should be examined for free haemoglobin. The presentation and figures given in this example are characteristic of paroxysmal nocturnal haemoglobinuria.

(*c*) The definitive test is Hamm's test. The red blood cells in paroxysmal nocturnal haemoglobinuria are more readily haemolyzed in acidified serum than are normal cells. Although the condition carries the term nocturnal, episodes of haemolysis are not necessarily overnight and haemoglobinuria is not found in one half of series of patients. The basic defect lies in the erythrocyte membrane which is sensitive to complement lysis although a specific defect has not been described.

Answer 7.3

(*a*) This patient had an iron deficiency anaemia as shown by the reduced MCV (microcytic cells), the reduced MCHC, the low serum iron and the increased iron binding capacity − normally about 30%.

(*b*) Some anaemia (9−11 g/dl) is common in rheumatoid arthritic patients and is usually normocytic and normochromic. Aspirin is a drug regularly used by these patients and causes mild but persistent blood loss.

(*c*) In this patient a different analgesic was then used and the haemoglobin gradually rose to 11 g/dl. The anaemia was thereafter refractory to oral and intramuscular iron so it was considered that the residual anaemia was that associated with rheumatoid arthritis.

Answer 7.4

(*a*) and (*b*) Thalassaemia minor and pyridoxine-responsive anaemia are the two most common explanations of this apparently refractory iron deficiency anaemia. In both disorders serum iron should be measured and the bone marrow examined. In both, the plasma iron is high and the marrow contains increased iron stores. Thalassaemia is diagnosed by electrophoresis of the haemoglobin. The pyridoxine-responsive anaemia is diagnosed by the response to oral pyridoxine in doses of up to 200 mg orally daily.

There are two further diagnostic possibilities, both rare. Firstly, a sideroblastic anaemia may have a hypochromic blood film. Secondly, there is a condition of congenital absence of transferrin. Here iron absorption is supranormal and an excessive iron is found in some tissues. The marrow is low in iron and the erythrocytes are hypochromic.

Answer 7.5

(*a*) This child had acute lymphoblastic leukaemia (ALL).
(*b*) He should be admitted to hospital for the following:

> (*i*) Bone marrow aspiration (the majority of cells are immature lymphocytes).
> (*ii*) Exclusion of infectious mononucleosis (Paul–Bunnell test) as this may produce similar clinical and blood changes.

(*c*) Admission is also necessary for the commencement of treatment which is in two stages. Firstly, remission is induced with drugs such as vincristine, asparaginase and prednisolone for a period of 6 weeks. This is followed by maintenance therapy with courses of vincristine, methotrexate and prednisolone, together with intrathecal methotrexate and prophylactic CNS irradiation to prevent CNS relapse. Therapy is continued for at least 3 years from remission.
(*d*) The five year survival is no better than 50% and of these some may still be on therapy because of relapses.

Answer 7.6

(*a*) The MCV is elevated (the limit of normal is 100 fl). The serum vitamin B_{12} is very raised and target cells (these are erythrocytes which have a well stained central area, then an intermediate pale zone and a well stained periphery) are present. These three features strongly suggest the anaemia of chronic liver disease. The explanation for macrocytosis in the presence of a normoblastic bone marrow and ample B_{12} is unknown.

(b) The next step in investigation of this man would be to examine his liver function. Indicated tests include: serum albumin, alkaline phosphatase, alanine aspartase (SGPT), bilirubin and perhaps liver biopsy.

Answer 7.7

This is an iron deficiency anaemia in a patient who had a treated B_{12} deficiency anaemia. The B_{12} deficiency is on the basis of an atrophic gastritis; these patients have an increased incidence of carcinoma of the stomach. Such tumours bleed and cause iron deficiency anaemias. The probable diagnosis was therefore carcinoma of the stomach.

Answer 7.8

(a) This patient had a moderately severe iron deficiency anaemia. All indices of circulating red blood cells are low as is the serum iron. The iron binding capacity is raised.

(b) The most likely cause would be secondary to heavy periods. Bleeding from the gut such as occurs from an ulcer is also common. Iron deficiency anaemia is quite frequent following pregnancies especially if they occur at short intervals. In a normal pregnancy about 750 mg of iron may be lost by the mother. A poor diet often is a contributory factor to any of the above causes.

Answer 7.9

This child either had haemophilia A (Factor VIII) deficiency or haemophilia B (Factor IX) deficiency (Christmas disease). He did not have a von Willebrand disease: in that condition the bleeding time is prolonged as well as the PTT.

To differentiate between haemophilia A and B, assays for specific factors must be conducted.

Answer 7.10

This man had both microcytes and macrocytes in the circulation at the same time. There are two reasons:

(*i*) The microcytes and the MCHC of 30 g/dl reflect a pre-existing iron deficiency anaemia as might have occurred from chronic blood loss from a duodenal ulcer.
(*ii*) The macrocytes are explained because after an acute bleed reticulocytes and normoblasts are seen in the peripheral film and both are larger than mature erythrocytes.

Answer 7.11

(*a*) The presence of myeloblasts in the peripheral blood film suggests that the patient had developed myeloid (myeloblastic) leukaemia as a complication or extension of his original polycythaemia. This occurs in about 25% of patients with polycythaemia rubra vera.
(*b*) The bone marrow is hyperplastic, the majority of cells being myeloblasts. The anaemia is consequent upon the leukaemic cells 'crowding out' the erythrocyte precursors.
(*c*) The prognosis is very poor, the average duration of survival from the time of diagnosis of this complication being only months.

Answer 7.12

(*a*) This man had polycythaemia rubra vera as shown by the raised haemoglobin, PCV and white blood cell count.
(*b*) Confirmation of the diagnosis is by demonstrating a red blood cell count of about $7-8 \times 10^{12}/l$ and that the red cell mass is increased to 40–94 mg/kg bodyweight (normal range 30 mg/kg bodyweight). The bone marrow is increased in extent and shows increased red blood cells, myeloid cells and megakaryocytes. Neutrophil alkaline phosphatase staining is increased. Marrow iron stores are depleted. Chronic bronchitis is the most common cause of secondary polycythaemia and should be excluded by clinical examination and lung function tests.
(*c*) Treatment includes venesection, [32] P, irradiation of the bone marrow or cytotoxic drugs.

Answer 7.13

(a) This is a leucoerythroblastic blood picture as shown by the presence of white blood cell precursors and nucleated red blood cells in the peripheral blood.

(b) Confirmation is obtained by examining a stained smear of bone marrow aspirate.

(c) The disease may be associated with bony deposits from cancer of the breast, bronchus, stomach or prostate. It is also found in myelofibrosis, chronic myeloid leukaemia, myeloma and polycythaemia rubra vera. Tuberculous infiltration of the bone marrow is uncommon in Western Europe but may produce a leucoerythroblastic blood picture and is a treatable condition.

Answer 7.14

(a) This child had thrombocytopenic purpura. Further investigation would show prolonged bleeding time and increased capillary fragility. The bone marrow would show an excess of early forms of megakaryocytes which stain badly and scanty platelet budding.

(b) Prednisolone is frequently used to suppress anti-platelet antibodies, not necessarily to control severe bleeding but to avoid the danger of an intracerebral bleed. Often prednisolone is only needed for a few weeks.

(c) In those few patients who relapse following prednisolone withdrawal, the liver and spleen should be scanned following intravenous administration of radio-labelled platelets. This may demonstrate the principal site of destruction. If this is the spleen, splenectomy will probably cure or ameliorate the condition.

Answer 7.15

(a) This woman had Addisonian megaloblastic anaemia (PA). The macrocytes and the hypersegmented neutrophils (PA polys) strongly suggest the diagnosis.

(b) The diagnosis should be proved by finding a low vitamin B_{12} concentration (less than 100 ng/l) (100 $\mu\mu$g/ml), a histamine-fast achlorhydria and defective radio-vitamin B_{12} absorption (Schilling test). Note that a bone marrow biopsy does not prove the diagnosis as it will only show non-specific megaloblastic changes.

(c) In Addisonian anaemia auto-antibodies to the cytoplasmic component of gastric parietal cells are found in 80% of patients, binding antibodies to intrinsic factor in up to 40% and blocking antibodies to intrinsic factor in 70% of patients. In addition auto-antibodies to other organs are frequently present — especially against the components of the thyroid glands.

Answer 7.16

A high platelet count of this degree may be found in the following:

(*i*) Chronic blood loss.
(*ii*) Post-splenectomy.
(*iii*) Polycythaemia rubra vera.
(*iv*) Myelosclerosis.
(*v*) Haemorrhagic thrombocythaemia. In this rare condition the platelets are morphologically abnormal and functionally defective. The spleen is often atrophic or absent.

Answer 7.17

(*a*) This infant had haemorrhagic disease of the newborn as shown by the normal coagulation indices with the exception of a prolonged prothrombin time.
(*b*) The treatment is intramuscular vitamin K which corrects the prolonged prothrombin time within a few hours. Occasionally a transfusion may be needed.

Other sites of bleeding include the gastrointestinal tract and the skin. The lesion is common in low birth weight babies. The present practice of giving vitamin K to all babies at birth, particularly those of low weight and of instrumental delivery, makes the condition now relatively unusual.

Answer 7.18

(*a*) Despite the negative Schilling test this patient has pernicious anaemia for three reasons:

(*i*) All the data are entirely compatible with this diagnosis.
(*ii*) The high titre of antiparietal cell antibodies is suggestive of this diagnosis.
(*iii*) Patients with ileal disease have an impaired ability to absorb vitamin B_{12} even in the presence of intrinsic factor — hence the negative Schilling test.

(*b*) Proof of pernicious anaemia in this patient could be obtained by measuring the reticulocyte count 5 to 8 days after the Schilling test (intramuscular vitamin B_{12}). A patient with pernicious anaemia responds maximally with a reticulocyte response between days 5 and 8.

Answer 7.19

(*a*) This man had an acquired primary sideroblastic anaemia. The features are a fairly severe anaemia with dimorphic red blood cells with a raised serum iron and normal or raised iron binding capacity.

(*b*) The marrow would show an increase in iron stores – a greater number and size of iron granules. In some marrow cells the iron granules form a peripheral ring in the cytoplasm: sideroblasts.

Answer 7.20

(*i*) Bone marrow examination.

(*ii*) The bone marrow should be stained for acid fast bacilli and cultured for these organisms.

(*iii*) A skeletal survey may show secondary tumour deposits from thyroid, breast, bronchus, stomach or prostatic tumours which would require further investigation. A skeletal survey might also show evidence of Paget's disease.

(*iv*) Lymph node biopsy would demonstrate Hodgkin's disease and plasma immunoglobulins may be abnormal.

(*v*) Urine testing for a Bence-Jones proteinuria may be indicated.

(*vi*) Iliac crest trephine biopsy may be performed if sternal puncture produced a dry tap and may lead to the diagnosis of myelofibrosis.

Answer 7.21

(*a*) The ECG is that of pulmonary hypertension. There is right axis deviation with a dominant S in lead I together with enlarged P waves (P pulmonale) and dominant R waves in the right chest leads.

(*b*) This may therefore be the ECG of cor pulmonale secondary to chronic bronchitis with a secondary polycythaemia. The ECG would also fit a pulmonary embolic or thrombotic episode which is a complication of primary polycythaemia.

Answer 7.22

This result is diagnostic of nothing. The second portion of the Schilling test would have to be performed – oral labelled vitamin B_{12} together with oral intrinsic factor. If the amount of radioactivity in the urine then increased this would be diagnostic of intrinsic factor deficiency and hence inability to absorb vitamin B_{12}. There are variations in the normal amount of labelled vitamin B_{12} which is collected in urine from laboratory to laboratory. Eleven per cent recovery is in the low normal range for most patients without vitamin B_{12} deficiency anaemia. For full interpretation of this patient's condition more information is necessary.

Answer 7.23

(a) 110–130 fl (μm^3).

(b) There will be depressed absorption of vitamin B_{12} with and without intrinsic factor.

(c) The bacteria which overgrow in the stagnant loop of bowel may synthesize folate which is absorbed and leads to supranormal serum concentrations.

(d) The upper small gut is normally sterile; a blind loop becomes colonized by large numbers of coliform and bacteroides species. The organisms compete for available vitamin B_{12} and may consume sufficient to produce a megaloblastic anaemia. Malabsorption of iron and products of digestion also occurs. The malabsorption of fat is caused by the splitting of bile salts by the blind loop bacteria into compounds which are toxic to the mucosa of the small gut.

In this patient there was a megaloblastic B_{12} deficiency anaemia with a mild iron deficiency component and steatorrhoea.

Answer 7.24

(a) Assuming that this patient had pernicious anaemia (that is failure to absorb vitamin B_{12} from the terminal ilieum) the most common explanation of failure of treatment is the co-existence of an iron deficiency anaemia.

(b) A megaloblastic marrow alone is not proof of a vitamin B_{12} deficiency. There may be a co-existence of folate deficiency, which may be dietary in origin or related to pregnancy or cirrhosis. Folate malabsorption may occur in bowel diseases or may be related to an anticonvulsant, folic acid antagonists (methotrexate) or use of the oral contraceptive.

This case illustrates the need for adequate investigations of a megaloblastic anaemia before any treatment is given.

Answer 7.25

(a) There was a thrombocytopenia but the normal marrow excludes idiopathic thrombocytopenic purpura. The rubella HAI titre was normal. Possibly his 'German measles' was some other viral infection since the clinical diagnosis is inexact.

(b) Thrombocytopenia may develop acutely following a viral infection.

(c) An assay of antiplatelet antibodies would be of value, because such antibodies may arise during a viral infection. In this boy they were not detected.

(d) No specific therapy is indicated, unless severe bleeding necessitates platelet transfusions. In the absence of antiplatelet antibodies, steroid therapy is of debatable value.

Answer 7.26

(*a*) From the information given the diagnosis was an obstructive jaundice and in a woman aged 62 years carcinoma of the pancreas is quite probable.

(*b*) The coagulation deficiency is likely to be secondary to vitamin K malabsorption which is frequent in obstructive jaundice. This is due to a lack of bile salts which are essential for the emulsification and hence absorption of fats and the fat soluble vitamins (A, D, K). In this patient two intramuscular doses of vitamin K resulted in a return to normal of the coagulation profile.

Answer 7.27

(*a*) The most likely diagnosis was Rhesus incompatibility between fetus and mother.

(*b*) The differential diagnosis involved both Rhesus and ABO incompatibilities.

(*c*) The further essential investigations were cord blood Coombs' test and the mother's blood and Rhesus group. If the cord blood was Coombs' positive then the infant had Rhesus incompatibility and the mother will be Rhesus negative. From the given data the degree of Rhesus incompatibility is mild as the haemoglobin is more than 12 g/dl and the bilirubin less than 68 μmol/l (4 mg/100 ml). If the cord blood was Coombs' negative then the diagnosis was an ABO incompatibility between mother and fetus and the maternal blood was very probably Group O. This is so because Group O incompatibility is much more common than any other blood group incompatibility.

Answer 7.28

The following imply poor prognosis: hypoalbuminaemia (secondary to renal loss), hypercalcaemia, a raised plasma creatinine (normal 60–140 μmol/l (0.68–1.9 mg/100 ml) and an IgA concentration more than 50 g/l (5.0 g/100 ml). A high MCV at presentation would probably be explained by folate deficiency arising from an increased folate demand by the tumour. As such this would imply a larger tumour mass than a 'normal' myeloma and would be expected to have a worse prognosis.

Favourable factors include: a normal haemoglobin, infrequent lytic lesions seen on skeletal survey and an IgG peak of less than 50 g/l (5.0 g/100 ml).

Non-prognostic factors given in this data include the tumour mass of 10^{12} cells/m^2 — this is the number of cells in an 'average' myeloma patient; urinary λ and χ chains are a feature of the disease and the urinary calcium can either be considered to be normal and hence good, implying no hypercalcaemia, or it may be reduced due to renal damage and therefore bad.

Answer 7.29

The answers to this question are most easily displayed in tabular form:

	Myelofibrosis	Chronic myeloid leukaemia
(i)	Tear-drop poikilocytosis characteristic Prominent anisocytosis	Usually normal
(ii)	Usually normal	Often more than 1000 ng/l ($\mu\mu$g/ml)
(iii)	Usually normal	Often much raised
(iv)	Absent	Usually present in 80% of cases
(v)	Normal to low	Normal to raised; falls as the disease progresses
(vi)	Normal or increased	Low or absent
(vii)	Often raised to 30–40 × 10^9/l (30–40 000/mm^3)	Usually more than 50 × 10^9/l; may reach 500 × 10^9/l (50–500 000/mm^3)
(viii)	May occur	Not reported

Answer 7.30

This child had kala-azar (leishmaniasis). The diagnosis was made by finding Leishman–Donovan bodies in the bone marrow. The features of bleeding, weight loss, enlarged abdomen (liver and spleen), anaemia (haemolytic), leucopenia with lymphocytosis and greatly raised IgG are all characteristic of the condition.

Answer 7.31

(a) It is unlikely that this child had leukaemia despite white blood cell precursors in the blood film as the platelet count was normal, there was an elevated reticulocyte count and marked abnormalities of the red blood cells — hypochromia, microchromia, poikilocytosis and target cells. This is a leucoerythroblastic blood picture but the major abnormality lies within the erythrocytes. This child had thalassaemia major in which abnormal peripheral white blood cells are found. The red blood cell findings in this case are characteristic and one would expect the haemoglobin to be in the region of 5–7 g/dl (g/100 ml) with a target cell count of 10–30% and a red cell count of $2-3 \times 10^{12}/l$ $(2-3 \times 10^6/mm^3)$.

(b) Children with thalassaemia major fail to thrive, are pale with enlarged spleen and liver and have 'mongoloid' facies.

(c) Haemoglobin electrophoresis would show various degrees of increased HbF and low or raised HbA_2. HbA may be absent.

(d) (i) The skull shows thickened diploë with thin outer and inner tables with perpendicular striae appearing between the tables leading to the 'hair-on-end' appearance.

(ii) In long bones, especially the distal ends of the femora, the medulla is increased and the cortex thinned. Short bones tend to be rectangular in contour with a trabeculated medulla giving a mosaic pattern.

Answer 7.32

(a) This man had an obstructive jaundice and Coombs' negative spherocytosis. The combination suggests a long-continued haemolytic anaemia with the development of bile pigment gallstones. Bile is present in the urine because of the obstructive jaundice. Spherocytes cannot be biconcave and have a normal volume; hence their diameter is less than normal. Osmotic fragility is increased.

(b) This man should be questioned regarding his antecedents. Hereditary (congenital) spherocytosis is an autosomal dominant and other members of his family would have had the condition. However this condition could arise as a mutation in the absence of a positive family history.

(c) The spleen was palpable.

Answer 7.33

(a) This nurse had liver cell damage, a haemolytic anaemia, raised serum IgM and a lymphocytosis with a neutropenia. Many of the lymphocytes were characteristic of infectious mononucleosis.

(c) Confirmation may be obtained by the heterophil antibody test (Paul–Bunnell) and by the demonstration of a rising titre of antibodies against the Epstein–Barr virus. All the abnormal laboratory findings quoted in this example may be found in a patient with infectious mononucleosis. Small epidemics of this condition occur from time to time in hospital staff.

Answer 7.34

From the data given it is clear that the child had a haemoglobinopathy. The positive metabisulphite test indicates the presence of HbS. However, target cells are not a feature of sickle-cell disease but are very frequently seen in thalassaemia. In sickle-cell disease some red blood cells have increased and some have decreased osmotic fragility. All the other data given in this question fit either diagnosis.

This child, who was of Mediterranean origin, had HbS, HbF and some HbA$_2$ upon electrophoresis and the resulting haematological features were of combined sickle-cell disease and thalassaemia.

Answer 7.35

(*a*) The blood urea was raised. A bicarbonate of 18 mmol/l is not unduly low for a child with diarrhoea and vomiting. A Hb of 10.2 g/dl (g/100 ml) is not unusual in a toddler. The platelet count was low and petichiae should suggest the diagnosis of meningococcal septicaemia but the platelet count would initially be normal.
(*b*) Low platelets and blood in the stools suggest haemolytic—uraemic syndrome.
(*c*) This is confirmed by a blood film showing burr cells and a raised reticulocyte count.
(*d*) The clinical course would likely be one of rapid deterioration, falling haemoglobin and rising blood urea with oliguria. Many cases are fatal but some recover with supportive therapy and/or heparinization.

ENDOCRINOLOGY

Answer 8.1

(*a*) This woman had Cushing's disease (pituitary-dependent bilateral adrenocortical hyperplasia due to excessive pituitary production of ACTH). This is shown by the suppression of plasma cortisol (and hence the excessive ACTH) by dexamethasone.

(*b*) The disease may be treated at either the adrenal or pituitary level. Bilateral adrenalectomy followed by maintenance cortisone is very effective. The pituitary can be irriadiated either externally or by an intrapituitary implant of yttrium 90. Metyrapone and/or aminoglutethimide, which interfere with cortisol synthesis, may be needed to supplement irradiation therapy or prior to bilateral adrenalectomy.

Answer 8.2

(*a*) This man had raised serum cortisol concentrations at 09.00 and 24.00 hours and after attempted dexamethasone suppression. He therefore had either an adrenal tumour (Cushing's syndrome) or atopic ACTH production. He did not have Cushing's disease (chromophobe or less frequently basophil, adenoma) because in this condition the ACTH feedback control while set at a supranormal level will be suppressed by dexamethasone.

(*b*) Two obvious reasons for weakness of the legs were either hypokalaemia (secondary to the renal effects of excess cortisol) or a proximal muscle myopathy. This is quite frequent in Cushing's syndrome.

Answer 8.3

(*a*) This girl had pseudohypoparathyroidism. If the facies were normal the differential diagnosis would include idiopathic hypoparathyroidism.

(*b*) Additional investigations include the following: (*i*) Parathyroid hormone (PTH) assay. PTH is found in the plasma but infusion of PTH has no phosphaturic effect nor does it increase urinary C AMP excretion. (*ii*) The hands should be X-rayed, as the metacarpals are shortened, especially the fourth and fifth.

(*c*) The face tends to be rounded and flat with a small bulbous nose and straight mouth; squints may be present.

The term pseudohypoparathyroidism is misleading as the defect is thought to be a lack of adenyl cyclase in the renal tubules and hence a failure to respond to PTH. The plasma biochemistry is that of secondary hypoparathyroidism. Pseudopseudohypoparathyroidism is a condition which is clinically identical to pseudohypoparathyroidism but the plasma biochemistry is normal.

Answer 8.4

(*a*) This woman had hypothyroidism. Almost always thyroid failure is associated with increased TSH levels except in pituitary or hypothalamic hypothyroidism when TSH is absent from the serum. The fact that this woman responded with a very brisk increase in plasma TSH indicates that she had tertiary (or hypothalamic) hypothyroidism. In secondary (pituitary) hypothyroidism there is a subnormal response of the serum TSH to the intravenous administration of TRH.

(*b*) With evidence of abnormal hypothalamic function the possibility of intracranial disease and possible hyposecretion of other pituitary hormones should be considered.

Answer 8.5

(*a*) This man had a raised GFR, together with hypercalcuria and raised plasma phosphate. These are all features of active acromegaly and his symptoms also fit the condition.

(*b*) The two essential additional investigations were:

(*i*) Measurement of an elevated plasma growth hormone (normally less than 10 ng/ml while at rest and fasting).

(*ii*) Demonstration of failure to suppress growth hormone (normally to below 5 ng/ml) during an oral glucose tolerance test.

Answer 8.6

(*a*) This man had the carcinoid syndrome.

(*b*) The diagnosis was established by measuring the urinary excretion of 5-hydroxyindole acetic acid (5-HIAA). Normal 24 hour excretion of 5-HIAA is about 2–10 mg; in the carcinoid syndrome usually more than 50 mg/day are excreted.

(*c*) Other features involve a transient hypotension with attacks of flushing, flushing induced by taking alcohol, pulmonary stenosis (and hence right heart failure), reversible airways obstruction leading to wheezing, abdominal discomfort, borborygmi and diarrhoea.

Answer 8.7

This is an example of hypercalcaemia and hyperthyroidism presenting together. This is a recognized although uncommon association. It is thought that the hypercalcaemia is explained by increased bone re-absorption. With treatment of the hyperthyroidism, hypercalcaemia ceases. If this does not occur then an alternative explanation of the hypercalcaemia has to be found.

Answer 8.8

(a) These findings indicate the presence of diabetes insipidus. The patient lost 3.5 kg in 8 hours and urine osmolarity remained low. There was therefore polyuria due to the absence of ADH. A normal response to fluid deprivation for 8 hours is a weight loss of less than 0.5 kg bodyweight and a rise in urine osmolarity to 700–1000 mmol/l.

(b) This man was known to have anterior pituitary failure and with cortisol treatment his ability to excrete water improved (as is usual) and nocturia developed. In addition to anterior pituitary failure he had posterior pituitary failure the features of which were masked by cortisol deficiency.

Answer 8.9

(a) This woman had panhypopituitarism as shown by subnormal levels of thyroxine, cortisol, glucose, ACTH, growth hormone and the failure of growth hormone to rise during deep sleep. The condition is also called Simmond's disease. Following a severe postpartum haemorrhage the condition is known as Sheehan's syndrome.

(b) Symptoms and signs may be vague but also include premature wrinkling of the skin and pallor (normochromic anaemia), loss of scalp, axillary and pubic hair and a general loss of secondary sex characteristics with atrophy of the breasts and genitalia. There may be headaches and visual impairment (optic chiasmal compression). The physical signs include bradycardia and hypotension.

Answer 8.10

This man had acromegaly as suggested by the increasing heel pad thickness. The remainder of his investigations indicated anterior pituitary failure – this is caused by progressive enlargement of an eosinophilic adenoma of the anterior lobe of the pituitary. Eventually the tumour led to a pituitary infarction and hence hypothyroidism, hypoandrogenism (normal plasma testosterone for men 9–24 mmol/l (0.320–1.0 µg/100 ml)), hypoadrenalism and the failure of growth hormone to rise under the stimulus of hypoglycaemia and TSH to increase after TRH. Panhypopituitarism is not an uncommon sequel of acromegaly.

Answer 8.11

(*a*) This electrolyte picture is entirely compatible with a diagnosis of Addison's disease or chronic hypoadrenalism. Hyponatraemia occurs because there is insufficient mineralocorticoid activity to permit the kidney to retain sodium adequately. The urinary sodium excretion rises disproportionately to dietary sodium and hyponatraemia occurs. In an attempt to compensate, the kidney retains an 'excess' of potassium and mild hyperkalaemia develops. The blood urea is usually normal as there is no significant impairment of the GFR.

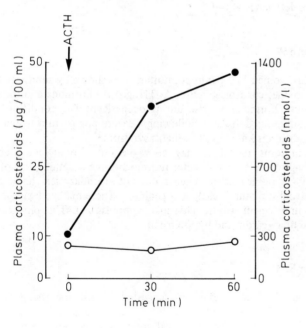

Figure 35

170

(*b*) Addison's disease is confirmed by demonstrating a failure of rise in plasma cortisol following intramuscular injection of synthetic ACTH (*Figure 35*). If plasma cortisol rises after ACTH an alternative explanation of the abnormal electrolytes must be found.

Answer 8.12

Cortisol production rate rises to about twice normal in Cushing's syndrome but may be increased by a factor of 10 if atopic ACTH is being secreted. A plasma ACTH of 280 pg/ml is very high; in Cushing's syndrome it rarely exceeds 200 pg/ml. The urinary 17-OHCS (17-hydroxycorticosteroid) excretion rises after metyrapone and falls after dexamethasone in Cushing's syndrome; no change is found after using these drugs in patients with atopic ACTH production. Blood sugar is raised in both conditions and does not aid in differentiation between the two diseases.

Answer 8.13

(*i*) Hyperthyroidism.
(*ii*) Fever.
(*iii*) Heart failure.
(*iv*) Phaeochromocytoma.
(*v*) Acute leukaemias.

The BMR is an estimation of oxygen consumption after overnight fasting. Under these conditions it is assumed that the respiratory quotient (RQ) is 0.85 and that the consumption of 1 litre of oxygen corresponds to the liberation of 20.22 kJ. In the five conditions listed above such patients are not in a basal state and oxygen consumption is therefore increased. Conversely the BMR is low in oedema and ascites, anorexia nervosa, malnutrition, hypoadrenalism and hypothermia.

Answer 8.14

The patient is euthyroid judged by the normal serum thyroxine and PBI. The high uptake of ^{131}I reflects secondary hyperplasia of the thyroid together with excess TSH which is secondary to the thyroid-blocking effect of carbimazole. In this state the gland is avid in iodine-trapping and hence an ^{131}I study does not give useful information. Success of antithyroid therapy should be judged clinically and supported by measurements of serum thyroxine.

Answer 8.15

This patient had fairly severe hyperthyroidism; all the investigations support the diagnosis. The T3 uptake test may lead to confusion as it can be reported in one of two opposite conventions. In the convention used here the reduced value indicates reduced free binding sites for circulating thyroxine as is found in hyperthyroidism or hypoproteinaemia. The T3 uptake test is thus not a measure of circulating triiodothyronine.

A hyperthyroid state may stem from a diffusely overactive gland (Graves' disease) or a toxic adenoma ('hot nodule'). Clinical examination may be able to differentiate between these two states and confirmation obtained by scintiscanning of the thyroid which will reveal specific adenomata. In Graves' disease the whole of the gland is supra-active on scanning and thyroid auto-antibodies are also present in the serum.

Answer 8.16

(a) This woman had myxoedema presenting with a carpal tunnel syndrome (myxoedematous compression of the median nerve at the wrist). Constipation and deafness (which is perceptive) are also recognized features of myxoedema.

(b) Pernicious anaemia is a condition caused by antiparietal cell antibodies and there is an overlap with thyroid disease which may also be mediated immunologically (antithyroid antibodies).

(c) Other features of myxoedema include: mental and physical sluggishness, cold intolerance, hypothermia, weight gain, croaking voice, dry and rough skin which may be yellowish and has a generalized non-pitting thickening of subcutaneous tissue, dry and brittle hair, menorrhagia, delayed relaxation of the tendon jerks, bradycardia, angina pectoris, peripheral cyanosis and Raynaud's phenomenon, 'depression' ('myxoedema madness').

Answer 8.17

(a) This was a lag type curve because the highest glucose concentration was found at 30 minutes and the concentration then fell below usual levels at 60 and 90 minutes. The insulin response is slow proportional to the blood glucose concentration and subsequently is 'excessive'.

(b) A lag curve may be found:

   (i) in post-gastrectomy and post-gastrojejunostomy patients in whom the glucose enters the small gut more rapidly than usual with consequent more rapid absorption.

(*ii*) in very severe liver disease, thought to be due to decreased glycogenesis.

(*iii*) occasionally in thyrotoxicosis presumably secondary to very rapid glucose absorption.

(*iv*) in apparently normal people – reactive hypoglycaemia.

Answer 8.18

(*a*) It was highly probable that this man had an oat cell carcinoma of the lung producing atopic ACTH and hence much increased (usually 2–10 times normal) plasma concentrations of cortisol. The renal effects of cortisol are sodium retention and compensatory excessive potassium loss. The hypokalaemia leads to an intravascular alkalosis (serum bicarbonate 33 mmol/l in this man). The glycosuria is explained by the diabetogenic effect of cortisol.

(*b*) The prognosis is very poor as an oat cell lung tumour is highly malignant and resistant to therapy. Those patients that have biochemical abnormalities at presentation frequently only have weeks to live.

Answer 8.19

(*a*) The chromatin positive buccal smear indicates the presence of two X chromosomes in a cell, i.e. a genotypic female. Only one X is active, the other is seen as a darkly staining spot at the periphery of the nucleus, the Barr body. In the case of a genotypic male, no Barr body is seen and the patient is chromatin negative.

The karyotype indicates the normal number of chromosomes for a female. The urinary ketosteroid excretion was within the normal range.

(*b*) (*i*) Pseudohermaphroditism. In female pseudohermaphroditism the phallus may be enlarged by exogenous steroids (progesterones given to the mother in the treatment of threatened abortion) or endogenous steroids in the adrenogenital syndrome, in which the urinary excretion of ketosteroids would be raised. This patient is basically female as indicated by the chromatin and karyotype and had ovaries.

In male pseudohermaphroditism by contrast, the gonads are testes, the karyotype is 46XY, chromatin negative but the external genitalia are intermediate and look basically female.

(*ii*) True hermaphroditism. The patient has both ovary and testis. The karyotype may be either male or female, chromatin positive or negative. Mosaicism has been described. Gonads may be palpable in the inguinal region or the labia.

(*iii*) Hypospadias with a bifid scrotum would be in the clinical differential diagnosis but buccal smear and karyotype exclude it in this example.

(*iv*) Simple labial fusion may occur in the female.

(*c*) If the gonads were palpable in the perineum, gonadal biopsy would be indicated together with laparotomy to define the pelvic anatomy.

Answer 8.20

(*a*) The clinical features might suggest Klinfelter's syndrome – but these patients have primary hypogonadism with decreased plasma concentration of testosterone (normal range 9–24 nmol/l). The increased prolactin concentration (normal range less than 10 μg/l in adult males) with the depressed plasma testosterone suggests a hypothalamic lesion.

(*b*) This man would therefore need:

(*i*) X-rays of the sella turcia;
(*ii*) investigations of the hypothalamic–pituitary axis;
(*iii*) visual field testing.

He was shown to have a pituitary tumour extending upwards and compressing the hypothalamus leading to hyperprolactinaemia.

Answer 8.21

This patient had a subnormal response to synthetic ACTH. This is very suggestive of therapeutically induced adrenal insufficiency secondary to prednisolone given to the patient during the survival of the transplanted kidney. A normal response to intramuscular synthetic ACTH is an increment in the 30 minute serum cortisol of at least 190 nmol/l (about 7 μg/100 ml) with the serum cortisol rising to at least 500 nmol/l (about 20 μg/100 ml). From the latter criterion this patient was in a subadrenal state.

Answer 8.22

(*a*) This woman experienced evening attacks of hypoglycaemia.

(*b*) This is a common feature in pregnant diabetics. Increased sensitivity to insulin occurs characteristically during the first trimester of pregnancy. The clinical picture may be confusing because glycosuria is not a feature of an ordinary hypoglycaemic episode. In this woman glycosuria represented the reduced renal threshold to glucose which is a normal feature of pregnancy.

IMMUNOLOGY

Answer 9.1

(a) This is an example of a Type I (immediate hypersensitivity as classified by Gell and Coombs) reaction in an atopic patient. The patient had extrinsic asthma.

(b) The reaction is mediated by specific IgE tissue antibody and mast cells when in contact with the antigen to which the individual is hypersensitive.

(c) The drug used to prevent this response was disodium cromoglycate (Intal) which in part is believed to prevent mast cells from degranulating and hence releasing vasoactive amines (histamine, 5-HT and slow releasing substance).

Answer 9.2

(a) Wiskott–Aldrich syndrome.

(b) Sex-linked recessive.

(c) Anaemia, thrombocytopenia, low serum IgM and IgG and a high IgA (normal ranges for this aged child, 0.5–2.0, 5–14, 0.5–1.8 respectively). There was also a low T-cell count (normal 470–1800 spontaneous sheep red blood cell rosettes/mm^3). The B-cell count was normal (range 200–1590/mm^3).

(d) Supportive treatment with antibiotics, blood and platelet transfusions are of limited benefit. Transfer factor has been used in some patients. Bone marrow transplant is probably the treatment of choice if a suitable donor can be found.

Answer 9.3

(a) The 'odd man out' disease is pernicious anaemia.

(b) All the other conditions are non-organ specific immune diseases while pernicious anaemia is an organ specific immune condition. In the non-organ specific diseases pathological changes are widespread and are primarily lesions of connective tissue, often with fibrinoid necrosis. Skin, muscle, renal glomeruli, joints, serous membranes and blood vessels are chiefly affected. Antinuclear antibodies are common in this group of diseases while antigastric mucosa antibodies are infrequent.

Pernicious anaemia, on the other hand, has auto-antibodies directed against the cytoplasmic component of gastric parietal cells in 80 to 90%

of patients and antibodies directed against nuclear protein in about 10%. There is a big overlap between pernicious anaemia and auto-immune thyroid disease; however these conditions are not mediated by cross-reacting antibodies but by two populations of antibodies which may be present in patients with either or both of these conditions.

Answer 9.4

(*a*) No. Group O patients' serum contains anti-A and anti-B. Such a transplant would be incompatible and a hyperacute rejection would occur.

(*b*) (*i*) Yes.
(*ii*) Yes.

There is no anti-red blood cell antigen in the serum of a patient with an AB genotype (group AB, phenotype). Other factors set aside, a success-ful transplant would be possible.

Answer 9.5

(*a*) Seropositivity in a patient with rheumatoid arthritis indicates that rheumatoid factor is detectable in the patient's serum.

(*b*) Rheumatoid factor is a specific IgM and IgG antibody directed against the patient's own IgG (antigen). The rheumatoid factor is synthesized in plasma cells within the synovium of affected joints and consists of auto-antibodies. Why such patients' immunoglobulins become immunogenic and induce the production of auto-antibodies is unknown.

(*c*) Weakness of dorsiflexion in a rheumatoid patient suggests the possibility of a peripheral neuropathy which develops in such patients. At age 67 years the possibility of a mild stroke has to be considered and it is also well recognized that in rheumatoid disease of the cervical spine the long tracts may be compressed. The foot should be examined for the Babinski response. If it is positive (extensor plantar) the lesion lies at the level of the cervical portion of the spinal cord or at the internal capsule. If there is no extensor plantar response then further examination of the foot may show other signs of a peripheral neuropathy.

Answer 9.6

(*a*) This patient had rheumatoid arthritis.

(*b*) This disease is characterized by an arthropathy associated in many patients with a positive rheumatoid factor (*see* Answer 9.5).

(c) These effusions are exudates as shown by their low albumin concentration. The high lymphocyte and eosinophil counts together with a low glucose concentration are characteristic of rheumatoid effusions.

(d) The differential diagnosis of the pleural effusion includes malignancy and tuberculosis as both can be associated with low glucose levels in the fluid. The abnormal cells in this patient were the so-called 'rheumatoid arthritis-cell' but initially suggested the possibility of cancer.

Answer 9.7

(a) This woman had nephrotic syndrome: oedema, hypo-albuminaemia and a proteinuria of more than 5 g daily.

(b) With a background of non-organ specific auto-immune disease it is possible that a similar disease process had developed — systemic lupus erythematosus with renal involvement. Alternatively renal amyloid, an occasional complication of Still's disease, may have developed. Renal damage secondary to long-continued analgesics should be considered but is excluded by the normal IVP and the nephrotic state. The nephrotic syndrome may be secondary to gold or penicillamine therapy in a patient with chronic joint disease.

(c) The antinuclear factor should be measured and a renal biopsy undertaken.

In this woman the ANF was not present and many glomeruli contained amyloid depositis. The amyloid was expected as λ and κ light chains were found in the urine. This is a feature of some patients with renal amyloid. The explanation is unclear but it is thought that during a long-continued inflammatory process excess immunoglobulin (antibody) is formed, some of the light chains of which are excreted in the urine. In other patients with amyloid a different protein (amyloid A) has been isolated. The full importance of these observations to clinical medicine is not yet known.

Answer 9.8

(a) The history is typical of polymyalgia arteritica (rheumatica) in which there was giant cell arteritis of the right temporal and ophthalmic arteries.

(b) The diagnosis is established by a biopsy of the tender superficial temporal artery (or other involved artery of the scalp or occiput).

(c) The condition is treated with prednisolone 40–60 mg daily.

(*d*) Treatment must be begun at once before the histological diagnosis is made. If treatment is delayed thrombotic occlusion of the involved arteries occurs which in this patient would have led to blindness of the right eye and necrosis of the area supplied by the superficial temporal artery. High dose prednisolone is continued until the ESR is normal and then very slowly reduced as the condition may relapse acutely.

Answer 9.9

(*a*) This child was an example of the Di George syndrome. This consists of aplasia of the thymus and parathyroid deficiency presumably due to malformation of the third and fourth branchial pouches. Lymphocytes which form spontaneous rosettes with sheep red blood cells are T-cells — lymphocytes which have been processed by the thymus to become immunologically competent and are then able to aid in defence against infection.

(*b*) Lymph node biopsy will show the bursa-dependent zones to be normally populated but the thymus-dependent zones (paracortical areas) will contain no lymphocytes.

(*c*) A fetal thymus graft alone will restore the immune system to normal in the Di George syndrome.

Answer 9.10

(*a*) The albumin and α_1-globulin peaks are reduced and there is an obvious increase in the gamma region with fusion of the beta and gamma regions.

(*b*) Assuming the electrophoresis was of serum the most likely diagnosis is cirrhosis, in which all the above features are found. The other possible diagnosis is nephrotic syndrome, but in this condition α_2-globulin is very frequently increased in concentration and the gamma globulin concentration is less frequently raised than in cirrhosis.

If the electrophoresis was of urine, the patient would have had a proteinuria of more than 15 g daily and this would have been of the non-selective type.

In clinical practice abnormal electrophoretic patterns of plasma or urine protein are usually of little or no help.

Answer 9.11

(*a*) The loci are on chromosome 6.

(*b*) Four subloci are recognized — D, B, C and A. Further ones will probably be described.

(c) Each locus is associated with a series of alleles (mutually exclusive genes). The sublocus B is the 'strongest' in antigenic (transplant rejection) terms. HLA 8 is on the B locus and it appears to occur more frequently in patients with coeliac disease, Graves' disease, Addison's disease, systemic lupus erythematosus, intrinsic asthma, dermatitis herpetiformis and juvenile diabetes mellitus.

Answer 9.12

This woman had mixed connective tissue disease. The history, high ESR and a positive ANF indicate an auto-immune state. The normal DNA binding and complement level exclude systemic lupus erythematosus. The speckled appearance of the ANF and the high titre of the anti-ribonuclear protein antibodies make the diagnosis.

This condition is amongst the connective tissue disorders and diagnosis is serological and not clinical. One advantage of establishing the diagnosis is to distinguish these patients from those with systemic lupus erythematosus. The prognosis in mixed connective tissue disease is probably better than that in systemic lupus erythematosus.

Answer 9.13

(a) There are four skin diseases in which immunoglobulins and complement are deposited in uninvolved areas: pemphigus, pemphigoid, lupus erythematosus and dermatitis herpetiformis.
(b) In about 60% of patients with dermatitis herpetiformis the small bowel shows villous changes identical to those found in coeliac disease. The intense pruritus of dermatitis herpetiformis responds within hours to oral dapsone.

Answer 9.14

Triple organ disease is not common: the most likely explanation of these figures in Western Europe would be amyloid of the so-called secondary type. Also included in the differential diagnosis are arteritides such as Wegner's granulomatosis, systemic lupus erythematosus and perhaps polyarteritis nodosa. Sclerodermia is a possible cause but liver involvement in this condition is infrequent although gut and kidney damage are well recognized.

Answer 9.15

The CH50, C4 and C3 titres are all depressed into the pathological range. This is compatible with classical pathway activation. It is also possible that both classical and alternative pathway activation are occurring together.

The complement cascade involves its nine components in the following order: C1, C4, C2, C3, C5, C6, C7, C8 and C9. Classical pathway activation proceeds from C1 to C9. Alternative pathway activation proceeds from C3 to C9 and does not involve C1, C4 and C2, the concentrations of which remain normal. Thus, if C3 is reduced in concentration while C4 is normal, alternative pathway activation is occurring. In this example, both classical and alternative activation may be present because as yet there is no test which will reliably indicate that activation of both pathways is occurring at the same time.

Answer 9.16

In a sense, none of the suggested investigations would be of much help as they are not measurements of the abnormalities which exist in Bruton's agammaglobulinaemia — namely failure of production of immuno-globulins.

All tests of the cellular immune response are normal, as is the circulating lymphocyte count. The diagnosis is made by demonstrating that very little immunoglobulin is present. Serum IgG is rarely above 10% mean normal adult concentration and IgA and IgM are less than 1% of mean normal adult concentrations.

Note that despite repeated infections, peripheral lymph nodes and tonsils are hypoplastic and may be absent.

Answer 9.17

(a) An MCV of 115 fl (μm^3) is well within the megaloblastic range and coupled with a jejunal biopsy indicates a probable malabsorbtive condition.

(b) The normal jejunum plasma cell population consists of mainly IgA synthesizing cells and a change to IgM predominance is seen in coeliac disease. Likewise in this condition serum IgM is decreased in about 60% of patients and there appears to be a higher incidence of isolated IgA deficiency when compared with a matched controlled population. Antireticulin antibodies may be demonstrated also in coeliac disease.

(c) There is an increased incidence of HLA B1 and B8 antigen in coeliac patients compared with control populations.

Answer 9.18

(a) This boy had developed a graft versus host reaction (GVHR). Such reactions occur in 70% of patients receiving a marrow transplant. The aetiology is obscure. The skin changes may be acute at 7 to 21 days after the transplant, or later within the first 6 weeks, with a diffuse reddening and scaling, lichenoid lesions or bullae. Diarrhoea and liver dysfunction may also be features.

(b) The following are the conditions under which GVHR may occur:

(i) The graft must have contained immunologically competent cells.
(ii) The host must contain transplant iso-antigens which are foreign to the graft.
(iii) The host must be incapable of mounting an effective immunological reaction against the graft.

Answer 9.19

(a) This man had a hyperviscosity syndrome on the basis of a Waldenstrom's macroglobulinaemia.
(b) Serum should be electrophoresed to demonstrate the much increased immunoglobulin peak and the IgM concentration quantitated.
(c) The fundi showed extremely dilated venules and multiple haemorrhages.
(d) Urgent plasmaphoresis is indicated to restore consciousness and preserve vision. Subsequently cytotoxic therapy is needed.

Answer 9.20

This is a Type III or soluble complex response and is mediated by both specific IgG antibody (and perhaps IgE) and complement. A Type I response (also called immediate or anaphylactic) develops a wheal and flare in a few minutes and subsides within 30 minutes. The Type I response is mediated by specific IgE (reagenic) antibody alone. A Type IV response (delayed hypersensitivity, Mantoux reaction) does not begin for at least 24 hours and may last 4 days. This skin test is mediated entirely by B-cells.

Answer 9.21

This woman had sclerodermia (progressive systemic sclerosis), affecting the hands and the oesophagus. The immunological investigations point to no specific diagnosis but the history is very suggestive of sclerodermia. While Raynaud's phenomenon is a fairly common condition sclerodermia develops in less than 2% of women with this vasomotor instability.

PHARMACOLOGY

Answer 10.1

Cephaloridine and gentamicin are both nephrotoxic and if given at too high a dose will cause renal failure and hence elevation of the blood urea and serum creatinine. Methylsergide, used for resistant cases of migraine, can lead to retroperitoneal fibrosis and if the ureters are involved, renal failure. Hypokalaemia is a side effect of many diuretics including bumetanide. An MCV of 109 is raised as in megaloblastic anaemia. Such an anaemia may complicate long-term trimethadione or azathioprine therapy. Trimethadione can act as a hapten and glomerular damage leading to proteinuria is recognized. Thrombocytopenia may follow the use of drugs including aspirin, phenylbutazone and azathioprine. High-dose aspirin also acts as a uricosuric agent and lowers serum urate levels.

Answer 10.2

(a) This man had Paget's disease (osteitis deformans) of the pubic rami and acetabulae. Also, as is common when bone close to large joints becomes pagetoid, osteoarthritis developed which contributed to the pain.
(b) The raised serum alkaline phosphatase and urinary hydroxyproline excretion reflect osteoblastic and osteoclastic activity respectively.
(c) If symptoms cannot be controlled with analgesics and non-steroidal anti-inflammatory drugs, a number of different agents are available. They include fluoride, glucagon, mithramycin, calcitonin and diphosphonates. The latter two are the most practical therapeutic agents. Either of these drugs will reduce elevated serum alkaline phosphatase and the urinary excretion of hydroxyproline. They should not be used unless these biochemical indices are raised. The ideal duration of therapy with either agent has not been adequately defined.

Answer 10.3

(a) Dependent oedema, hypo-albuminaemia and hypercholesterolaemia strongly suggest the presence of a nephrotic syndrome. With the reduced creatinine clearance it is highly probable that the glomeruli will show obvious damage when examined microscopically.
(b) The past history of this woman is typical of that of Familial Mediterranean fever. At least 30% of patients with this condition develop renal amyloid which was demonstrated in this patient.

(c) The major drugs of use in nephrotic syndrome are spironolactone (to ameliorate secondary hyperaldosteronism) and a 'loop' diuretic to initiate and subsequently, at lower dosage, to maintain the patient relatively oedema free.

Colchicine is of value in preventing the attacks of abdominal pain in Familial Mediterranean fever and may also prevent the development or progression of amyloid.

Answer 10.4

(a) The symptoms and high urinary catecholamine levels suggest either a phaeochromocytoma or the rebound phenomenon which occurs in some patients who withdraw their regular doses of clonidine abruptly.

(b) This man had left his supply of clonidine at home. The explanation of this phenomenon is not known but it is believed that during clonidine treatment there is increased storage of catecholamine in nerve terminals by the stimulation of inhibitory α-receptors. If the drug is suddenly stopped the stored amines are released, producing phaeochromocytoma-like symptoms, and their urinary excretion increases.

(c) In the acute phase probably the treatment of choice is clonidine – symptoms subside rapidly and blood pressure is lowered. Alternatively labetalol may be used which has α- and β-blocking properties and can also be given parenterally.

Answer 10.5

(a) This man had hyperosmolar non-ketotic diabetic coma (HNC) as shown by the grossly elevated blood glucose, the hypernatraemia and the absence of ketones.

(b) The osmolality by calculation was 393 mmol/l (for details of calculations *see* Answer 6.8, page 142).

(c) Patients with HNC are severely dehydrated with marked hypernatraemia and hypokalaemia. Therapy includes the following:

(i) Hypotonic saline (77 mmol/l, 0.45%).

(ii) Relatively larger quantities of potassium than needed in a patient with keto-acidosis.

(iii) Relatively small doses of insulin.

(iv) Very frequent biochemical reassessment.

(v) Despite the severe dehydration, fluid replacement should be less rapid than in keto-acidosis. This reduces the risk of cerebral oedema and allows serum osmolality to fall to normal gradually.

The mechanism of HNC is not adequately understood; it tends to occur in, and even may be the presentation of, maturity onset diabetes. Thiazides and diazoxide are both diabetogenic and apparently act as initiating factors.

Answer 10.6

(a) These data were obtained from a man with respiratory failure.

(b) He had been given oxygen at too high a concentration. This is shown by the greatly raised Pco_2 of 141 mmHg (18.8 kPa). Respiratory failure is diagnosed in a chronic bronchitic if Po_2 is less than 60 mmHg (8.0 kPa) and Pco_2 is more than 49 mmHg (6.5 kPa). A person in respiratory failure breathing air cannot have a Pco_2 above 80 mmHg (10.6 kPa) in order for the Po_2 to be compatible with life.

(c) Apart from chest deformities associated with long-standing bronchitis, this man was semiconscious, not coughing, not cyanosed and had papilloedema.

(d) Further treatment is urgent and ideally involves transfer to an intensive care unit. Inspired oxygen in a concentration of 24% should be given, the patient roused and forced to cough during hourly physiotherapy. Intubation and aspiration of lung secretions may also be needed.

Answer 10.7

(a) This patient had osteomalacia.

(b) He returned with hypercalcaemia and the reduced alkaline phosphatase gave evidence of healing of the osteomalacia.

(c) A high dose of vitamin D is necessary in the presence of renal failure as the hydroxylation of D_3 to active metabolites of the vitamin is severely impaired in chronic renal failure. The follow-up interval was too great; the patient should have been seen at 2–3 weekly intervals to measure plasma calcium and to reduce the dose of vitamin D accordingly. The calcium × phosphate product from the second portion of the data is 10.5 if the measurements had been reported in SI units or 130 if reported in conventional units.

(d) Calcification in blood vessels around joints and the limbus may be demonstrated.

Answer 10.8

(a) This girl had acute on chronic renal failure as shown by the high urea (patients with urea in the 60 mmol/l (400 mg/100 ml) region tend not to have stable renal failure), the haemoconcentration and low urine volume accompanied by low urinary osmolality.

(*b*) Immediate management involves:

   (*i*) The central venous pressure line.
   (*ii*) Intravenous sodium chloride.
   (*iii*) Intravenous frusemide as the central venous pressure begins to rise towards normal.

(*c*) It is very probable that tetracycline had been prescribed for acne. This drug if given to patients in renal failure produces a brisk rise in blood urea with rapid clinical deterioration.

Answer 10.9

The two most likely compounds are either paracetamol (acetaminophen) or carbon tetrachloride as both may produce combined renal and hepatic failure. A third possibility is phenol or one of its derivatives. Glycerol poisoning may produce a similar picture but with both these latter compounds death is likely to occur before 4 days.

Answer 10.10

(*a*) The child was given oxygen at increasing concentrations. While the hyperoxaemia was relieved a dangerous hypercapnoea was induced with a consequent intense respiratory acidosis (pH 6.97).
(*b*) At this stage the child was unconscious and scarcely breathing.
(*c*) She was therefore intubated and at first, intermittent positive pressure respiration was used with an inspired oxygen concentration of 28%. Consciousness returned and assisted respiration using a Bird respirator from +9 to +14 hours was used while the inspired oxygen concentration was reduced to normal. At 14 hours after the admission extubation was successful.

Answer 10.11

(*a*) This woman had accelerated (malignant) hypertension. The normal urine microscopy and IVP virtually exclude primary renal disease. High concentrations of circulating renin are usually found in accelerated hypertension and are thought to be a reflection of renal damage secondary to the high pressure rather than a primary phenomenon.
(*b*) The increase in plasma renin is to be expected: frusemide causes renin release secondary to the sodium depletion it produces. Diazoxide causes renin release as a result of the increase in circulating volume consequent upon the peripheral vascular dilatation it produces. A fall in

GFR after aggressive hypotensive therapy is also to be expected; with stabilization of the blood pressure the GFR usually returns to, or may rise above, the pretreatment level.

(c) Diazoxide is a very potent hypotensive drug but has two important side-effects: intense sodium retention and a diabetogenic action. All patients taking diazoxide should receive a potent 'loop' diuretic and also a hypoglycaemic agent. Without these drugs the patient taking diazoxide will very probably develop hyperosmolar non-ketotic diabetic coma.

Answer 10.12

(a) This woman had gradually become digoxin intoxicated as indicated by the plasma digoxin of 2.7 ng/ml, and the rapid pulse was shown to be due to a mixture of atrial fibrillation and ventricular ectopic beats. Generally patients with plasma digoxin levels above 2.0 ng/ml are prone to develop digoxin poisoning.

(b) Renal function judged by blood urea and plasma creatinine is normal for this woman's age. About 35% of total body digoxin is excreted daily and its excretion is approximately proportional to creatinine clearance. However for either blood urea or plasma creatinine to rise the GFR has to be reduced by about 50%. Hence, in this woman, despite apparently normal renal function, the GFR had gradually fallen (due to senile nephron loss and perhaps renal emboli from the left atrium) and her dose of digoxin slowly became inappropriately high. It was found subsequently that 0.0625 mg of digoxin daily was adequate.

Answer 10.13

(a) This patient had a respiratory alkalosis consequent upon tachypnoea with wash-out of carbon dioxide.

(b) This was due to direct stimulation of the respiratory centre by salicylates. Initially renal excretion of bicarbonate will bring the pH back towards normal, producing a compensated respiratory alkalosis.

(c) Subsequently (in the absence of treatment) a combined respiratory and metabolic acidosis develops due to the following:

(i) Increasing concentration of salicylate depresses the respiratory centre and induces carbon dioxide retention (respiratory acidosis).

(ii) Renal function becomes impaired because of hypotension and dehydration with retention of organic metabolic acids.

(iii) Salicylates impair carbohydrate in metabolism with accumulation of acetoacetate, lactic and pyruvic acid.

(iv) Salicylate and its metabolites are acidic and further enhance the metabolic acidosis.

Answer 10.14

This is an example of interaction between clofibrate and warfarin. Both are protein bound and as some of the binding sites for warfarin were already occupied by clofibrate disproportionately severe anticoagulation occurred. The prothrombin time was found to be 75 seconds with a control of 15 seconds although the doses of warfarin given were correct in proportion to the weight of the patient.

Answer 10.15

(a) This patient had a megaloblastic anaemia in the presence of a normal serum B_{12} concentration. Megaloblastic anaemia appears only in a deficiency of B_{12} or folic acid. Some severe psoriatic patients need methotrexate to control their skin condition. Methotrexate binds to dihydrofolate reductase thereby blocking folate metabolism and producing megaloblastic anaemia.

(b) The anaemia must be treated with folinic acid and not by folic acid (pteroylglutamic acid). Folinic acid is already reduced and is beyond the metabolic step blocked by folic acid antagonists.

Answer 10.16

(a) The child was febrile but meningitis was excluded by the normal CSF. The urea is mildly raised and the bicarbonate depressed; hence some degree of dehydration was likely. Diabetes was excluded by the normal CSF sugar.

(b) Cerebral trauma is unlikely with the normal CSF but the skull should be X-rayed in this circumstance. The blood pressure should be measured. Poisoning should be suspected in unexplained unconsciousness and blood taken for salicylate assay (which would fit with the urea and bicarbonate concentrations) and for barbiturate assay. Serum should be kept to be examined for the presence of other drugs if further enquiry into the history indicates the necessity. Unconsciousness could also be postictal and an EEG might be helpful.

Answer 10.17

(a) The bile in the urine together with hyperbilirubinaemia and raised alkaline phosphatase indicate obstructive jaundice.

(*b*) A man with familial hypercholesterolaemia and raised triglycerides would be receiving treatment with clofibrate. One of the mechanisms by which this drug reduces plasma cholesterol is by increasing the excretion of cholesterol into the bile. The development of cholesterol stones is a complication of clofibrate therapy as in this patient.

Answer 10.18

(*a*) Lithium. Hypothyroidism with hypercalcaemia are recognized complications of lithium therapy.
(*b*) Also described are: nephrogenic diabetes insipidus, possible exacerbation of psoriasis, mania, reversible T-wave flattening and interaction with haloperidol leading to prolonged extrapyramidal symptoms.

Answer 10.19

(*a*) This patient had anticonvulsant osteomalacia.
(*b*) The condition is quite widely recognized in patients who need to take long-term anticonvulsants in large doses, in particular phenytoin and phenobarbitone.
(*c*) It is thought that non-specific hepatic induction by the anticonvulsant impairs vitamin D_3 hydroxylation with an increase in more polar inactive metabolites. There was therefore less 25-OHD$_3$ to be further hydroxylated to 24, 25-di-OHD$_3$ and 1, 24, 25-tri-OHD$_3$. The physiological function of 1, 24, 25-tri-OHD$_3$ is to promote gut absorption of calcium. In the presence of inadequate 1, 24, 25-tri-OHD$_3$ plasma calcium falls and eventually bone calcium becomes inadequate and osteomalacia develops.

In chronic biliary cirrhosis similar vitamin D metabolic abnormalities may develop and osteomalacia may occur.

Answer 10.20

(*a*) These changes in urinary excretion of urate, magnesium, calcium and iodide are induced by the thiazide group of drugs. The mechanism for urate, calcium and magnesium is not understood. Extra iodide is excreted because one of the properties of thiazides is that of chloruresis. Diuretics that produce chloruresis fail to modify the discriminatory function of the renal tubule for different halides.
(*b*) Acute gout is occasionally precipitated by thiazides due to retention of urate. Thiazides also have a diabetogenic effect.

(*c*) The ability to reduce calcium excretion with thiazide diuretics is of value in idiopathic hypocalcuria. Urine calcium may fall by as much as one-third with bendrofluazide and this property is used to augment other measures in reducing calcium excretion and hence stone formation in these patients.

Answer 10.21

The phenytoin level is below the therapeutic range (usually 3–16 mg/l) while the phenobarbitone concentration is modestly elevated (therapeutic range 4.0–4.2 mg/l). Two factors may account for the phenytoin levels. The patient may not be taking the dose prescribed or the dosage may not have been increased relative to the child's weight, if he has been on the drug over a number of years. The phenobarbitone level may be associated with hyperactivity and distractibility.

Answer 10.22

(*a*) This man had been treated with stilboestrol or a similar compound with oestrogen activity. These drugs cause the gynaecomastia by their oestrogenic side effect and oedema by renal sodium and hence water retention by their mineralocorticoid effect.
(*b*) If gynaecomastia is unacceptable orchidectomy is an alternative treatment but this is psychologically unattractive to some patients.

Answer 10.23

(*a*) The overnight urine osmolarity is low; in the absence of renal disease figures above 700 mmol/l are usual.
(*b*) This man had mild diabetes insipidus. It is now well recognized that lithium has an effect on water metabolism and it is thought that 10–15% of patients taking this drug develop diabetes insipidus of nephrogenic origin.

Answer 10.24

(*i*) Contraindicated: tetracycline, spironolactone and nitrofurantoin.
(*ii*) Relatively contraindicated: clofibrate, digoxin, metoclopramide, cephaloridine and ampicillin. A plasma creatinine of 256 μmol/l (2.9 mg/100 ml) implies a GFR of about 15–20% of normal and

hence retention of these drugs or their metabolites which are renally excreted is probable. These drugs should not be used therefore, or used in less frequent doses and plasma levels should be measured.

The other drugs mentioned in Question 10.24 may be used in conventional dosage.

Answer 10.25

A was adrenaline; B was dopamine; C was noradrenaline. These are the three naturally occurring sympathomimetic amines.

For a full explanation of these changes a textbook of pharmacology should be consulted; however it is clear that dopamine is a preferable pressor agent to noradrenaline in clinical conditions.

Answer 10.26

No precise diagnosis can be made from the data given. There is no reason to think that this woman had Conn's syndrome (primary hyper-aldosteronism) because:

(*i*) the plasma aldosterone was in the normal range;
(*ii*) while she was mildly hypokalaemic there was no accompanying alkalosis which is almost invariable in Conn's syndrome;
(*iii*) spironolactone will reduce the blood pressure to normal in cases other than those who have Conn's syndrome.

Answer 10.27

All are best avoided. Tetracycline is less well absorbed if given with either iron or aluminium hydroxide. Cholestyramine (which possesses anion exchange properties) impairs gut absorption of phenylbutazone as does phenobarbitone reduce the gut uptake of griseofulvin. PAS may reduce the serum concentration of rifampicin as some formulations of PAS contain betonite (a kaolin-like substance), present in the PAS granules, which binds rifampicin in the gut, reducing absorption.

Answer 10.28

The correct analysis to apply would be the Chi squared test to calculate the test statistic χ^2. This test is probably the most frequently used significance test in medical statistics. As the observations can be grouped according to two criteria a 2 × 2 contingency table can be drawn up:

	No. of mice surviving	No. of deaths
Treatment	21	3
No treatment	0	24

$\Sigma\chi^2 = 37.3$ and the number of degrees of freedom for a 2 × 2 contingency table is $\nu = 1$. From tables for the critical values of χ^2 when $\nu = 1$ and $P = 0.01$, $\chi^2 = 6.64$. The difference between the observed and expected events (death of mice) indicates that the null hypothesis is rejected and the probability that the 21 mice that survived have been treated with the cephalosporin is statistically significant ($P < 0.01$).

Answer 10.29

(a) Drugs that may have been used include α-blockers (phentolamine or phenoxybenzamine), diazoxide, hydrallazine, sodium nitroprusside, pentolinium or the α- and β-blocker, labetalol. A parenteral hypotensive agent that would not have produced such a dramatic response is clonidine, as an initial pressor (α agonist) effect may occur. A further drug which might produce a sudden fall in blood pressure is saralosyn which is a relatively specific blocker of angiotensin II.

(b) The high renin concentration may be of diagnostic value and suggests accelerated or renovascular hypertension but would not be of value in selecting a particular hypotensive drug.

(c) If the blood pressure fall had occurred following 5–10 mg of pentolamine the data would constitute a positive Rogitine test and would be suggestive of a phaeochromocytoma. However, false positives occur especially in uraemia and the diagnosis of a phaeochromocytoma rests upon circulating concentrations of adrenaline and noradrenaline and their excretion products and not a sudden depressor effect following intravenous α-blockade.

Answer 10.30

Each of these drugs possesses antithyroid activity and is goitrogenic. They all appear to impair the iodination of tyrosine and to affect the conversion of iodotyrosines to the active forms of thyroid hormone.

Lithium decreases the rate of hormone secretion from the gland and slows hormonal degradation. It should be emphasized that carbimazole and methylthiouracil are the only two drugs in this group which possess potent antithyroid acitivty. Hypothyroidism is only infrequently seen during prolonged courses of the other drugs.

Answer 10.31

This patient had a megaloblastic anaemia and steatorrhoea. This anaemia commonly accompanies chronic liver disease and perhaps reflects hepatic inability to store vitamin B_{12}. Steatorrhoea occurred following the increased neomycin dosage. Neomycin causes steatorrhoea by two mechanisms: it produces reversible and modest gut mucosal damage and also combines with bile and fatty acids leading to disruption of micelles. Malabsorption and hence increased faecal fat excretion occur.